PRACTICAL PROBLEMS in MATHEMATICS

for HEALTH OCCUPATIONS,

Second Edition

Delmar's *PRACTICAL PROBLEMS in MATHEMATICS* Series

- *Practical Problems in Mathematics for Automotive Technicians, 6e*
  Sformo, Sformo, and Moore
  Order # 1-4018-3999-1
- *Practical Problems in Mathematics for Carpenters, 7e*
  Huth & Huth
  Order # 0-7668-2250-8
- *Practical Problems in Mathematics for Drafting and CAD, 3e*
  John C. Larkin
  Order # 1-4018-4344-1
- *Practical Problems in Mathematics for Electricians, 6e*
  Stephen L. Herman
  Order # 0-7668-3897-8
- *Practical Problems in Mathematics for Electronic Technicians, 6e*
  Stephen L. Herman
  Order # 1-4018-2500-1
- *Practical Problems in Mathematics for Graphic Communications, 2e*
  Ervin A. Dennis
  Order # 0-8273-7946-3
- *Practical Problems in Mathematics for Health Occupations, 2e*
  Louise Simmers
  Order # 1-4018-4001-8
- *Practical Problems in Mathematics for Heating and Cooling Technicians, 4e*
  Russell B. DeVore
  Order # 1-4018-4177-5
- *Practical Problems in Mathematics for Industrial Technology*
  Donna Boatwright
  Order # 0-8273-6974-3

- *Practical Problems in Mathematics for Manufacturing, 4e*
  Dennis D. Davis
  Order # 0-8273-6710-4
- *Practical Problems in Mathematics for Masons, 2e*
  John E. Ball
  Order # 0-8273-1283-0
- *Practical Problems in Mathematics for Welders, 4e*
  Schell and Matlock
  Order # 0-8273-6706-6
- Practical Problems in Mathematics for Emergency Services
  Thomas B. Sturtevant
  Order # 0-7668-0420-8

Related Titles

- *Fundamental Mathematics for Health Careers, 3e*
  Hayden and Davis
  Order # 0-8273-6688-4
- *Diversified Health Occupations, 6e*
  Louise Simmers
  Order # 1-4018-14-565
- *Health Science Career Exploration*
  Louise Simmers
  Order # 1-4018-5809-0
- *Introduction to Health Science Technology*
  Louise Simmers
  Order # 1-4018-112-80

PRACTICAL PROBLEMS in MATHEMATICS

for HEALTH OCCUPATIONS,

Second Edition

Louise Simmers, MEd, BSN

THOMSON

DELMAR LEARNING

Australia   Canada   Mexico   Singapore   Spain   United Kingdom   United States

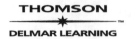

THOMSON
™
DELMAR LEARNING

Practical Problems in Mathematics for Health Occupations, Second Edition

Louise Simmers, MEd, BSN

Vice President, Technology and Trades SBU:
Alar Elken

Editorial Director:
Sandy Clark

Acquisitions Editor:
James Gish

Development:
Marissa Maiella

Marketing Director:
Dave Garza

Marketing Coordinator:
Mark Pierro

Production Director:
Mary Ellen Black

Production Manager:
Andrew Crouth

Library of Congress Cataloging-in-Publication Data
Simmers, Louise.
   Practical problems in mathematics for health occupations / Louise Simmers.— 2nd ed.
   p. cm. — (Delmar's practical problems in mathematics series)
   ISBN 1-4018-4001-9
   1. Nursing—Mathematics—Problems, exercises, etc. 2. Medicine—Mathematics—Problems, exercises, etc. I. Title. II. Series.
   RT68.S56 2005
   513'.1'02461—dc22
                              2004009553

NOTICE TO THE READER

Publisher does not warrant or guarantee any of the products described herein or perform any independent analysis in connection with any of the product information contained herein. Publisher does not assume, and expressly disclaims, any obligation to obtain and include information other than that provided to it by the manufacturer.

The reader is expressly warned to consider and adopt all safety precautions that might be indicated by the activities herein and to avoid all potential hazards. By following the instructions contained herein, the reader willingly assumes all risks in connection with such instructions.

The publisher makes no representation or warranties of any kind, including but not limited to, the warranties of fitness for particular purpose or merchantability, nor are any such representations implied with respect to the material set forth herein, and the publisher takes no responsibility with respect to such material. The publisher shall not be liable for any special, consequential, or exemplary damages resulting, in whole or part, from the readers' use, or reliance upon, this material.

Contents

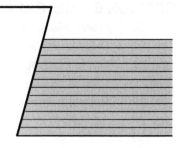

Preface

Practical Problems in Mathematics for Health Occupations, Second Edition, has been written to provide students with experience in computing problems that are common in a wide variety of careers in health care. Every health care occupation has mathematical concepts that must be learned. This book will provide students with examples of the many types of problems that may be encountered. At the same time, it will provide students with information about a wide variety of health care careers. In addition, terminology and abbreviations used in health occupations are incorporated throughout the book.

At the start of each unit, an introductory section provides a basic explanation of the concepts necessary to complete the problems in the unit. Examples are presented to help the learner review the mathematic principles. The problems in each unit progress from basic examples of the math concept to more complex examples that require critical thinking. As the student progresses through each unit, the student will become more proficient at solving a wide variety of math problems.

Two special units included in this textbook are the units on health care careers and medical abbreviations. The Careers in Health Care unit provides a basic introduction to more than 200 different health care careers. A brief description of the career, basic educational requirements for the career, and levels of workers in the career cluster are provided to allow the student to explore a wide variety of jobs in health care. The Common Medical Abbreviations unit provides a reference to interpret medical language. The abbreviations included are used in almost every health care career.

At the end of the book, an appendix and glossary provide additional assistance to both the instructor and student. The appendix contains a wide variety of conversion charts. The glossary provides technical and mathematical definitions to aid the student in learning terminology used in health occupations. Finally, answers to odd-numbered problems are found at the end of the book.

An Instructor's Guide is available for use with this workbook. It provides the instructor with answers to all of the problems in the workbook. It also contains two achievement reviews that can be used to effectively measure student progress.

Practical Problems in Mathematics for Health Occupations, Second Edition, can be used for a wide range of students at both the secondary and post-secondary level. For students with limited mathematical ability, additional instructor guidance will allow the student to master the concepts presented. For students with more advanced mathematical ability, the workbook can serve as a self-taught unit that allows the student to review basic math concepts and master more advanced concepts. Students can progress at their own rate and develop confidence as they complete each unit.

After completing all of the units in this workbook, students will have a strong foundation in required mathematics, a greater comprehension of many different health care careers, and knowledge about terminology and abbreviations used in health occupations.

ABOUT THE AUTHOR

Louise Simmers received a BS in Nursing from the University of Maryland and an MEd in Education from Kent State University. She has worked as a public health nurse, medical-surgical nurse, coronary care nurse, instructor of practical nursing, and as a diversified health occupations and anatomy and physiology instructor and school-to-work coordinator at Madison Comprehensive High School in Mansfield, Ohio. She has received the Vocational Educator of the Year Award for Health Occupations in the State of Ohio, and the Diversified Health Occupations Instructor of the Year Award for the State of Ohio. She is the author of other Delmar textbooks, *Diversified Health Occupations, Introduction to Health Science Technology,* and *Health Science Career Exploration,* that are used in many health occupations programs throughout the United States.

ACKNOWLEDGMENTS

The author would like to thank her husband, Floyd Simmers, a mathematics and precision machining instructor, who evaluated and solved all of the problems in this book. She would also like to thank all the editors at Delmar Learning and the reviewers who provided valuable input into the contents of this book. Without their help, the book would not have been written.

Delmar Learning and the author would like to thank the following reviewers for their valuable suggestions and technical expertise:

Tom Chartier
Woodbury Central High School/Western Iowa Tech Community College
Iowa

Diane M. Zimmerman, RN
Cape May County Technical High School
Cape May Court House, New Jersey

Kay C. Cornelius
Sinclair Community College
Dayton, Ohio

Joan M. Wolf, RN, MS
Buckeye Career Center
New Philadelphia, Ohio

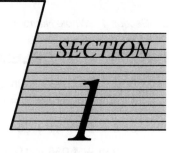

Whole Numbers

SECTION 1

Unit 1 *ADDITION OF WHOLE NUMBERS*

BASIC PRINCIPLES OF ADDITION OF WHOLE NUMBERS

Whole numbers refer to complete units with no fractional parts. Addition is the process of adding two or more numbers together to find an answer called a *sum*. Whole numbers are added by placing them in a vertical column with the numbers aligned on the right side of the column. The right column of numbers is added first. The last digit of the sum obtained is written in the answer. The remaining digit is carried to the next column and added to the numbers in that column. The process is repeated until all of the columns have been added in a right to left order.

Example: Find the sum of 33 + 549 + 6 + 878 + 75:

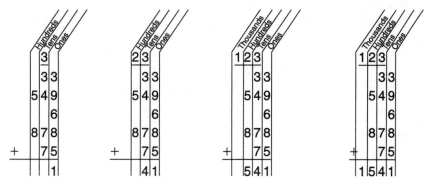

PRACTICAL PROBLEMS

1. Add the following numbers to obtain the correct sum. (*Hint:* Remember to align the numbers in a vertical column.)

   a. $8 + 25 + 11 + 356 + 19 =$ _____

   b. $238 + 4,056 + 19 + 586 + 1,039 + 77 =$ _____

   c. $128 + 4,700 + 25 + 9,215 =$ _____

   d. $993 + 5,687 + 63,921 + 94 + 7 =$ _____

   e. $1,003 + 5,791 + 536 + 88 + 4 =$ _____

   f. $8,849 + 919 + 729,648 + 596 =$ _____

2. Following is the time card for a physical therapy technician. How many hours did he work?   _____

DAY OF WEEK	HOURS WORKED
Sunday	0
Monday	8
Tuesday	11
Wednesday	7
Thursday	9
Friday	10
Saturday	5

3. A medical assistant (MA) must inventory all supplies every month. After checking the examination rooms, she counts the following numbers of oral thermometers: 7, 11, 13, 21, and 6. What is the total number of oral thermometers?   _____

4. The MA also counts the examining gloves in each room and determines that there are 331, 193, 82, 419, 206, and 73 gloves. What is the total number of gloves?   _____

5. A veterinary technician (VT) purchases a new uniform for her job. She buys a uniform for $67, shoes for $51, support hose for $7, and a name pin for $6. What was her total cost? (*Hint:* If a number represents specific units such as dollars, grams, pounds, or similar items, the symbol the number represents should be included in the answer. For example: $38, 431 gm, or 33 lb.)   _____

6. A worker in the obstetrical department of Children's Hospital creates a graphic chart showing the number of Caesarean sections (C-sections) performed per month. What is the total number of C-sections performed for the year?   _____

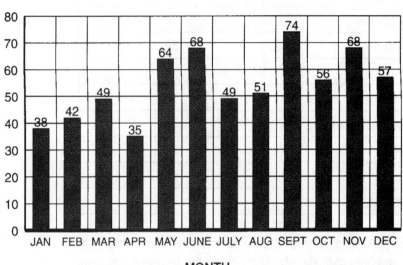

CAESAREAN SECTIONS

7. A registered nurse (RN) in a coronary care unit determines that one patient has been given the following intravenous (IV) solutions in a 24-hour period: 740 milliliters (ml) of 0.9% normal saline, 475 ml of Ringer's lactate, 1,250 ml of 5% dextrose in water, and 45 ml of an antibiotic solution. What is the total number of milliliters of IV solution the patient received?   _____

8. A dental assistant (DA) orders the following supplies: composite for $103, amalgam capsules for $386, alginate for $15, lab plaster for $55, stone for $89, and rubber base impression material for $54. What is the total cost of the order?   _____

9. A registered dietitian (RD) creates the following chart to show the amount of cholesterol in an average meal. What is the total amount of cholesterol in milligrams (mg)?   _____

FOOD	CHOLESTEROL (mg)
1 Fried Chicken Breast	238
¼ Cup Chicken Gravy	3
1 Cup Egg Noodles	53
¾ Cup Broccoli	0
1 Bran Muffin with Pat of Butter	11
½ Cup Coleslaw with Dressing	5
¾ Cup Ice Cream	45
1 Cup 2% Milk	18
TOTAL	

10. A geriatric assistant (GA) at a long-term care facility must encourage Mr. Berry to drink large amounts of fluids. Mr. Berry drank the following amounts of liquids: 260 cubic centimeters (cc), 355 cc, 80 cc, 125 cc, 65 cc, 240 cc, 145 cc, and 75 cc. What is the total fluid intake that should be recorded for Mr. Berry?   _____

11. The geriatric assistant must also calculate the urinary output of Mr. Berry. Mr. Berry voids the following amounts of urine: 335 cubic centimeters (cc), 265 cc, 180 cc, 245 cc, and 290 cc. What is the total urinary output that should be recorded for Mr. Berry?   _____

12. A statistician at a health department compiles the following 10-year graph to show the number of acquired immune deficiency syndrome (AIDS) cases in the state. What is the total number of AIDS cases for the 10-year period?   _____

AIDS CASES

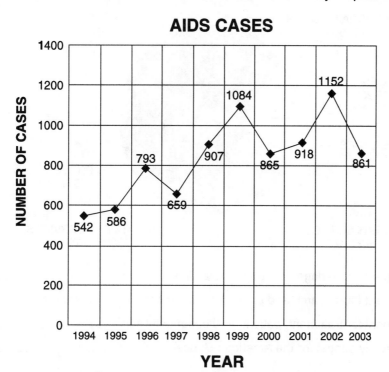

13. A student enrolled in a health occupations course learns that a diet should not contain large amounts of salt and that the recommended daily amount is 1,100 to 3,300 milligrams (mg). He decides to see how many mg of sodium are in a typical fast-food meal. His research reveals the following amounts of sodium: 1 bowl chili: 980 mg, 1 cheeseburger: 1,044 mg, 1 order of french fries: 224 mg, 1 milkshake: 299 mg, and 1 apple pie: 325 mg. How many milligrams of sodium does the meal contain?   _____

14. A pharmacy technician inventories the number of medication containers. She finds there are 1,139 safety-lock capsule containers, 978 easy-open capsule containers, 403 15-ml bottles, 1,256 30-ml bottles, and 285 ointment containers. What is the total number of medication containers?   _____

15. A volunteer for the American Cancer Society studies the following pie chart showing the yearly budget.

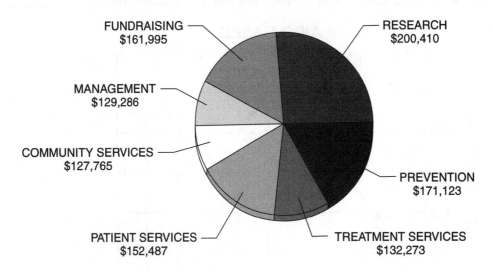

FUNDRAISING
$161,995

RESEARCH
$200,410

MANAGEMENT
$129,286

COMMUNITY SERVICES
$127,765

PREVENTION
$171,123

PATIENT SERVICES
$152,487

TREATMENT SERVICES
$132,273

a. What amount is spent for management and fundraising? _____

b. What amount is spent for research and prevention of cancer? _____

c. What amount is spent for treatment, patient, and community services? _____

d. What is the total yearly budget for the American Cancer Society? _____

16. The following chart shows the total number of runs made by Central City's Emergency Services. Complete the chart by calculating the total runs for each department for the third quarter and the total runs for each month of the quarter.

CENTRAL CITY EMERGENCY SERVICES
2004 THIRD QUARTER REPORT

Services	July	August	September	TOTALS
Fire Department	167	273	139	d.
Emergency Medical—EMS	486	537	515	e.
Rescue Squad	42	76	59	f.
TOTALS	a.	b.	c.	g.

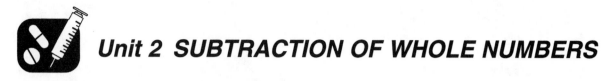 **Unit 2 SUBTRACTION OF WHOLE NUMBERS**

BASIC PRINCIPLES OF SUBTRACTION OF WHOLE NUMBERS

Subtraction is the process of finding the *difference*, or *remainder*, between two numbers or quantities. The number to be subtracted (subtrahend) is placed under the number from which it is to be subtracted (minuend) with both numbers aligned on the right side. Starting at the right side, subtract the bottom number from the top number.

Example:

Subtract 435 from 679:

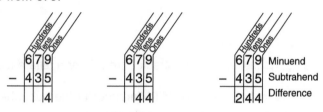

If the number being subtracted is larger than the number it is to be subtracted from, borrow 1 number from the digit to the left and add ten to the number that is too small. Then subtract 1 from the digit used for borrowing before using it to subtract the number below it.

Example:

Subtract 289 from 942:

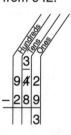

Because 9 is greater than 2, borrowing is required. 4 can be written as 3 tens plus 1 ten. Borrow 1 ten to increase the 2 to 12, leaving 3 tens. 9 can now be subtracted from 12 for a difference of 3.

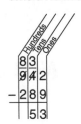

Because 8 is greater than 3, borrow 1 hundred from the 9 hundreds, leaving 8 hundreds. 8 can now be subtracted from 13 for a difference of 5.

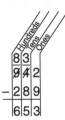

Because 2 is less than 8, borrowing is not necessary. 2 is subtracted from 8 for a difference of 6.

Hint: An easy way to check the answer is to add the answer (difference) to the subtrahend (number subtracted). If you get the minuend (original number), your answer is correct.

PRACTICAL PROBLEMS

1. Subtract the following numbers to obtain the difference.
   (*Hint:* Remember the simple way to check your answer.)

   a. $869 - 583 =$ _____

   b. $23,431 - 14,652 =$ _____

   c. $92,345 - 12,001 =$ _____

   d. $86,500 - 4,678 =$ _____

   e. $605,002 - 73,594 =$ _____

   f. $1,521,367 - 82,589 =$ _____

2. A diet consultant in a weight loss clinic has a client who weighed 203 pounds before starting the clinic's program. The client's current weight is 185 pounds. How much weight has the client lost? _____

3. A pediatric assistant is checking one-year-old Brian. His head circumference measures 45 centimeters (cm). At birth, his head circumference measured 37 cm. How much did Brian's head grow in one year? _____

4. A medical assistant (MA) must order supplies to keep the correct amount in stock. His inventory number and required number in stock are shown in the following chart. How many of each item must he order?

ITEM	NUMBER TO KEEP IN STOCK	INVENTORY NUMBER	AMOUNT TO ORDER
File Folders	2500	1386	
Folder Labels	3000	1892	
Prescriptions	250	189	
History Forms	5000	3045	
Data Sheets	5000	1098	

5. A certified nurse assistant (NA) gets overtime pay for all hours over 40 hours per week. In one month, she works 50 hours the first week, 47 hours the second week, 53 hours the third week, and 44 hours the fourth week. How many overtime hours did she work for the entire month?   _____

6. A patient care technician (PCT) in a coronary care step-down unit checks a patient's radial pulse (P) and it is 89. He then checks the patient's apical pulse (AP) and it is 167. What is the patient's pulse deficit? (*Hint:* A pulse deficit is the difference between the AP and the P.)   _____

7. A pharmacist is paid $53,921 per year. After a raise, her yearly salary increases to $56,059. What was the amount of her raise?   _____

8. A registered dietetic technician (DTR) is preparing a menu for a patient who is on a sodium-restricted diet that limits the sodium to 1,800 milligrams (mg) per day. He lists the patient's food intake and sodium content for breakfast and lunch on a chart. How many mg of sodium can the patient have for dinner?   _____

FOOD ITEM	MILLIGRAMS (mg) OF SODIUM
1 Bowl Raisin Bran Cereal	365
1 Cup 2% Milk	122
1 Glass Orange Juice	2
Fish Sandwich with Tartar Sauce	615
1 Bag Potato Chips	188
¾ Cup Frozen Yogurt	90
1 Diet Soft Drink	72

9. A medical accountant is calculating the bill for the Brian Nartker family. The original bill for medical services and minor surgery was $2,865. Mr. Nartker's insurance company sends a payment check for $1,938. Mrs. Nartker's insurance company sends a payment check for $479. How much do Mr. and Mrs. Nartker still owe?   _____

10. A geriatric assistant (GA) is calculating a resident's oral intake to record on an Intake and Output (I & O) record. The resident drank a partial glass of milk containing 240 cubic centimeters (cc). There were 152 cc left in the glass. How much did the resident drink?   _____

11. A nurse assistant (NA) has a patient positioned in a high Fowler's position with the patient's upper body elevated at a right angle. He is told to position the patient in a low Fowler's position with the patient's upper body at a 25° angle. How many degrees must he lower the patient's head? (*Hint:* Determine the number of degrees in a right angle.)

_____

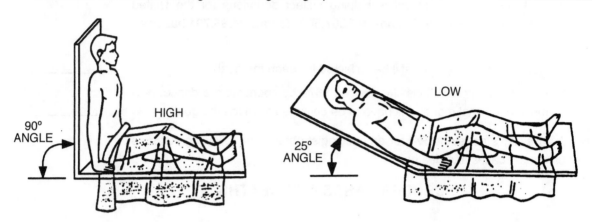

12. A student in a health occupations statistics course is studying statistics on acquired immune deficiency syndrome (AIDS) from the Centers for Disease Control and Prevention (CDC). The statistics show a total of 816,149 patients with AIDS. Of this number, 467,910 patients have died. How many patients are still alive?

_____

13. A dental hygienist (DH) is evaluating the average biting forces on the teeth as shown on the chart.

TYPE TEETH	POUNDS	NEWTONS (N) (1 lb = 4.44 N)
Molars	129	573
Bicuspids	72	320
Cuspids	51	226
Incisors	39	173

a. What is the difference in biting force in pounds between the molars and incisors?

_____

b. What is the difference in biting force in Newtons (a metric unit for measuring force) between the molars and cuspids?

_____

c. Which two types of teeth have the greatest difference in biting force in Newtons?

_____

14. A medical laboratory technologist (MT) notes that a patient's leukocyte (white blood cell or WBC) count before an appendectomy (surgical removal of the appendix) was 18,654. Two days after the appendectomy, the patient had a leukocyte count of 8,986. What was the drop in the leukocyte count?   _____

15. A health occupations student is helping collect donations for the United Appeal in her community. The goal is $357,500. To date, $286,791 has been raised.

   a. How much money must still be collected to reach the goal?   _____

   b. If her health occupations class raises $579 by sponsoring a dance, how much additional money will have to be collected to reach the goal?   _____

16. A physician's assistant (PA) for an oncologist obtains the following statistics on cancer cases and deaths.

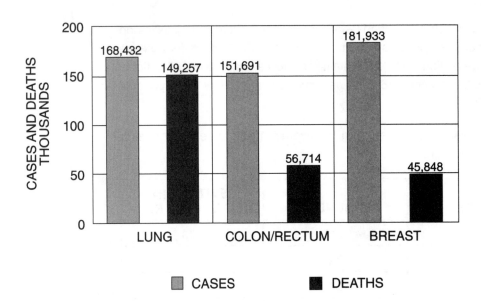

CANCER CASES AND DEATHS

   a. How many people with lung cancer lived?   _____

   b. How many more people died from lung cancer than breast cancer?   _____

   c. How many people lived after having one of the three types of cancer shown?   _____

Unit 3 MULTIPLICATION OF WHOLE NUMBERS

BASIC PRINCIPLES OF MULTIPLICATION OF WHOLE NUMBERS

Multiplication is actually a simple method of addition. For example, if three 7s are added, the answer is 21. If the number 7 is multiplied by 3, the answer or *product* is equal to 21. Therefore, $7 + 7 + 7$ is the same as 3×7.

$$\begin{array}{r} 7 \\ 7 \\ +7 \\ \hline 21 \end{array} \qquad \begin{array}{r} 7 \\ \times 3 \\ \hline 21 \end{array}$$

To multiply numbers, write the number to be multiplied, or the *multiplicand*, first. If possible, it is best to use the larger of the two numbers as the multiplicand. The product of 645×25 is the same as the product of 25×645, but it is easier to use 645 as the multiplicand. Under the multiplicand, write the number of times it is to be multiplied, or the *multiplier*, aligning the two numbers on the right side. Every number in the multiplicand is then multiplied by every number in the multiplier. If the product is greater than 9, the digit above 9 is carried to the next column to the left and added to the product of that column. The product for each multiplier is aligned under the multiplier, moving from right to left. When the second or successive multipliers are used, the product obtained is aligned under that multiplier, again moving from right to left. After all of the multipliers are used, the products obtained are added together to get the final product.

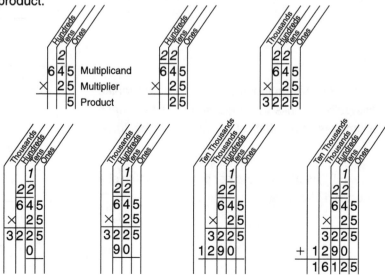

PRACTICAL PROBLEMS

1. Complete the following multiplication table.

0	1	2	3	4	5	6	7	8	9
1	1								
2		4							
3			9						
4				16					
5					25				
6						36			
7							49		
8								64	
9									81

2. Multiply the following numbers to obtain the correct product. (*Hint:* Remember to use the larger number as the multiplicand or top number.)

    a. $43 \times 287 =$ _____

    b. $236 \times 4,059 =$ _____

    c. $286 \times 300 =$ _____

    d. $572 \times 6,008 =$ _____

    e. $863 \times 70,804 =$ _____

    f. $9,654 \times 33,472 =$ _____

3. A geriatric assistant (GA) must record his patient's oral intake on an Intake and Output (I & O) record. His patient drinks three glasses of juice. If each glass contains 240 cubic centimeters (cc), what total oral intake should be recorded?   _____

4. A respiratory therapy technician (RTT) works 8 hours per day. One month she works 27 days. How many hours did she work that month?   _____

5. A medical laboratory technician (MLT) notes that it takes 30 milliliters (ml) of broth and 15 ml of agar to fill one agar slant tube.

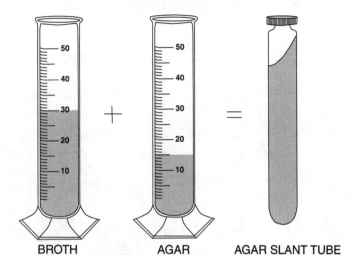

BROTH   AGAR   AGAR SLANT TUBE

a. How much broth would he need to fill 25 tubes?   _____

b. How much agar would he need to fill 25 tubes?   _____

6. A dental laboratory technician (DLT) uses 200 grams (gm) of stone for each dental model. How many gm of stone will she need to make 19 models?   _____

7. A student in an anatomy and physiology (A & P) course learns that the bones that make up the fingers and toes are called phalanges. Each thumb and great toe has two phalanges. All other fingers and toes have three phalanges each. What is the total number of phalanges a person has?   _____

8. A respiratory therapist (RT) is using a microscope to examine a sputum specimen. If the eyepiece on the microscope has a power of 15× (× means times; a power of 15× magnifies object 15 times) and the objective has a power of 40×, what is the total number of times she is magnifying the specimen? (*Hint:* To find total magnification on a microscope, multiply the power of the eyepiece times the power of the objective.)   _____

9. An electrocardiographic (ECG) technician examines the following six-second strip of an electrocardiogram she has recorded on a cardiac patient. How many times per minute is the patient's heart beating? (*Hint:* There are 10 six-second periods in one minute.) _____

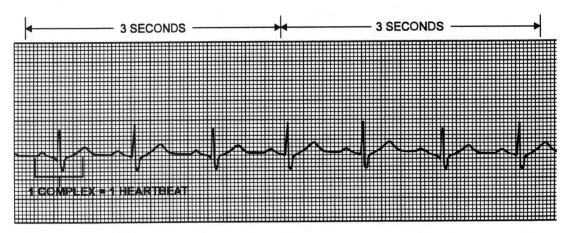

10. A registered nurse (RN) is giving a patient 250 milligrams (mg) of Tetracycline six times a day. How many mg of Tetracycline is he giving the patient per day? _____

11. A worker at Tiny Tot Child Care Center is preparing infant formula. There are 13 infants in the center and each infant drinks 5 ounces (oz) of formula six times per day. How many oz of formula must she prepare per day? _____

12. A student studying to be a cardiologist learns that the heart pumps about 65 milliliters (ml) of blood every time it beats. She checks her own pulse and finds her heart is beating 72 times per minute.

    a. How many ml of blood does her heart pump per minute? _____

    b. How many ml of blood does her heart pump per hour? _____

    c. How many ml of blood does her heart pump per day? _____

13. A worker in a weight loss clinic is calculating the number of calories needed by his clients. He knows that if a person is moderately active, the person should consume 15 calories per pound of body weight. If a person is active, the person should consume 20 calories per pound of body weight. He creates a chart showing the client's name, ideal body weight based on height, and degree of activity. Calculate the calories needed by each of the individuals shown on the chart.

CLIENT	IDEAL WEIGHT	ACTIVITY	CALORIES NEEDED
Tara Beers	157 pounds (lb)	Moderate	
Michelle Harod	134 lb	Active	
Floyd Smith	209 lb	Moderate	
Pat Brewster	128 lb	Moderate	
Terry Webel	165 lb	Active	

14. A pharmacist receives a prescription order from a physician. The physician wants the patient to take 40 milligrams (mg) of Furosemide qid (four times a day) for a period of 30 days. The pharmacist has 40-mg Furosemide tablets.

a. How many tablets should the pharmacist give to the patient for the 30-day period? _____

b. What is the total number of mg of Furosemide the patient will take in a 30-day period? _____

15.   A medical secretary maintains the accounts and writes the paychecks for a medical office complex. There are 36 people on the payroll. Eight people earn $7 per hour, eleven people earn $11 per hour, four people earn $13 per hour, six people earn $16 per hour, and seven people earn $23 per hour. If everyone works 40 hours per week, what is the total amount of money needed for the payroll each week?   _____

A DAY IN THE LIFE OF A TEENAGER

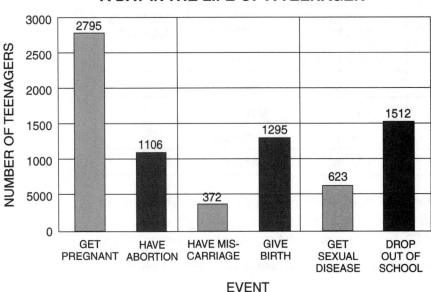

Note: Use the previous chart to answer questions 16–18.

16.   How many teenagers get pregnant each year? (*Hint:* Note that the figures on the chart are for one day. Do not calculate a leap year.)   _____

17.   How many teenagers get a sexually transmitted disease (STD) each year?   _____

18.   How many teenagers have an abortion or miscarriage each year?   _____

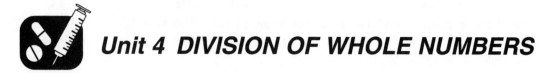

Unit 4 DIVISION OF WHOLE NUMBERS

BASIC PRINCIPLES OF DIVISION OF WHOLE NUMBERS

Division is a simplified method of subtracting a smaller number from a larger number many times. The number to be divided is called the *dividend*. The number used to indicate the number of times the dividend is to be divided is called the *divisor*. The answer is called a *quotient*. If the divisor cannot be divided into the dividend an even number of times, the number left over is called a *remainder*.

To begin the process of division, the dividend is placed inside the division bracket, the divisor is placed to the left of the dividend, and the quotient is placed above the dividend.

$$\text{Divisor} \overline{)\text{Dividend}}^{\text{Quotient}}$$

Calculate the number of times the divisor can be divided into the first number or numbers of the dividend. Since a divisor cannot be divided into a number that is smaller, the digits used in the dividend must represent a number larger than the divisor. Put this calculated number in the quotient, aligned directly above the last number used in the dividend. Multiply the divisor by this quotient and place the product under the dividend. If the product is larger than the dividend, a smaller number must be used as the calculated quotient. Subtract this product from the numbers used in the dividend. Check to make sure that the difference is less than the divisor. Then bring down the next number in the dividend and place it at the end of the number obtained when the product was subtracted. Now calculate the number of times the divisor can be divided into this new number. Again, place the answer in the quotient, multiply this number of the quotient times the divisor, place the product under the number, and subtract to obtain the difference. Continue this process until all numbers in the dividend have been used. Remember that each time you bring down a number, you must put a number in the quotient, even if the number is zero.

Example: Division without a remainder

Find the quotient of 3,614 ÷ 26.

```
      1            1            13           13           139
26)3614    26)3614     26)3614      26)3614      26)3614
   26          26           26           26           26
   ──          ──           ──           ──           ──
   10         101          101          101          101
                            78           78           78
                            ──          ───          ───
                            23          234          234
                                                     234
                                                     ───
                                                       0
```

Note: To check your answer, multiply the quotient by the divisor. If a remainder is present, add the remainder to the product. The final product should equal the dividend if your answer is correct. For example: 26 × 139 = 3614.

Example: Division with a remainder

Find the quotient of 779 ÷ 36.

$$
\begin{array}{r}
2 \\
36\overline{)779} \\
72 \\
\hline
5
\end{array}
\qquad
\begin{array}{r}
2 \\
36\overline{)779} \\
72 \\
\hline
59
\end{array}
\qquad
\begin{array}{r}
2\,1 \quad \text{R23} \\
36\overline{)779} \\
72 \\
\hline
59 \\
36 \\
\hline
23
\end{array}
$$

Note: Check your answer by multiplying the quotient by the divisor: 36 × 21 = 756. The answer had a remainder of 23 so this must be added to the product: 756 + 23 = 779. Since the final answer is the same as the dividend, the answer is correct.

PRACTICAL PROBLEMS

1.   Divide the following numbers to obtain the correct quotient.

   a. 1,554 ÷ 37 =   _____

   b. 5,063 ÷ 21 =   _____

   c. 756 ÷ 7 =   _____

   d. 3,939 ÷ 39 =   _____

   e. 26,325 ÷ 251 =   _____

   f. 75,483 ÷ 538 =   _____

2.   A dietetic technician (DT) knows his patient is allowed 729 calories of fat per day and that there are 9 calories per gram (gm) of fat. How many gm of fat can his patient eat per day?   _____

3.   A medical assistant (MA) orders 15 new stethoscopes for $555. How much did he pay for each stethoscope?   _____

4. A worker for a pharmaceutical supply company has 828 boxes of a lice treatment kit. She packages the boxes in cases for shipment to suppliers. How many cases does she ship to suppliers?   _____

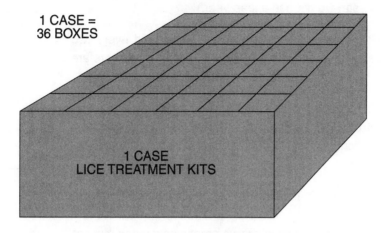

1 CASE =
36 BOXES

1 CASE
LICE TREATMENT KITS

5. Mr. Johnson has a heart attack and spends five days in the coronary care unit. His bill is $9,395. How much was he charged per day?   _____

6. A licensed practical nurse (LPN) gives a patient 1,800 milligrams (mg) of Streptomycin in a 24-hour period. How many mg does he give the patient per dose if he gives the medication q4h (every 4 hours)?   _____

7. A medical laboratory technician (MLT) has a flask containing 225 milliliters (ml) of a diluting solution. She must transfer the solution to 5-ml graduated pipettes. How many pipettes will she fill with the solution?   _____

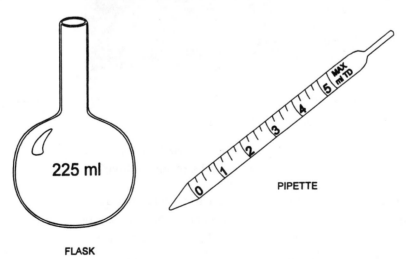

225 ml

PIPETTE

FLASK

8. A volunteer for the American Cancer Society sees statistics that show that approximately 526,695 people die each year in the United States from some type of cancer. How many people die of cancer each day? (*Hint*: Determine the number of days per year. Do not use a leap year.)   _____

9. A physical therapist (PT) makes $56,082 per year. He is paid every two weeks. What is his gross pay per paycheck? (*Hint:* Remember that there are 52 weeks per year.)   _____

10. A microbiologist is staining bacterial slides. She uses a bottle of acetone-alcohol decolorizer that contains 90 milliliters (ml) of solution. If each test requires 18 ml of the solution, how many tests can she perform with the bottle of solution?   _____

11. A patient care technician (PCT) knows that his patient's water pitcher contains 1,125 cubic centimeters (cc). His patient drinks the water out of a glass that contains 225 cc. If the water pitcher is empty, how many glasses of water did the patient drink?   _____

12. A dentist is evaluating different brands of amalgam capsules. She studies the label of one brand.

> **50 Capsules**
>
> ## AMALGALOY PREMIUM CAPS
>
> **TOTAL NET WEIGHT**
> **20,000 mg Alloy**
> **23,500 mg Mercury**

a. How many milligrams (mg) of alloy does each capsule contain?   _____

b. How many mg of mercury does each capsule contain?   _____

13. The gross pay per week of a respiratory therapist (RT) is $798. He works 6 days per week for 7 hours each day. How much does he make per hour?   _____

14. A student doing a report for his health occupations class learns that 9,525 people died of heart disease at a local hospital. The cost of health care for these people before their deaths was $258,365,625. If the same amount was spent for each person, what was the cost per person for health care?   _____

15. A dietitian is calculating the number of grams (gm) of fat in a fried shrimp dinner. He knows the dinner has a total of 847 calories (cal) and contains 18 gm of protein and 88 gm of carbohydrates. He also knows that there are 4 cal in one gm of protein, 4 cal in one gm of carbohydrates, and 9 cal in one gm of fat. How many gm of fat does the shrimp dinner contain?   _____

16. A sterile supply worker at a city hospital packages infectious waste for pick-up by the local garbage company. When the waste is in boxes, she has 15 boxes of one size, and 1 box that is the next size smaller. The total cost for removal of the boxes is $712. The cost for removal of various size boxes is shown on the chart.

SIZE OF BOX	COST PER BOX
2 Cubic Foot Box	$28
3 Cubic Foot Box	$37
4 Cubic Foot Box	$45
5 Cubic Foot Box	$56

a. What size boxes were used for the 15 boxes of infectious waste?   _____

b. What size box was use for the 1 smaller box of infectious waste?   _____

Unit 5 COMBINED OPERATIONS WITH WHOLE NUMBERS

BASIC PRINCIPLES OF COMBINED OPERATIONS

Many math problems involve more than just addition, subtraction, multiplication, or division of whole numbers. In many cases, two, three, and even all four of these operations are used to solve a single problem. This section will provide practice at solving problems that require the use of two or more of the operations.

A standard order must be followed when dealing with combined operations. The steps to follow include:

- *Do all operations inside parentheses first:* For example, in the problem $(8 - 3) \times 4 =$, the first step would be to subtract 3 from 8. The different of 5 would then be multiplied by 4 to obtain an answer of 20.

- *Solve any expressions that contain exponents or roots:* For example, in the problem $4^2 - (6 + 2) =$, the first step would be to add the 6 and 2 to obtain the sum of 8. The second step would be to square the 4, which means 4×4 for a product of 16. The third step would be to subtract the 8 from 16 to obtain an answer of 8.

- *Multiply or divide from left to right:* For example, in the problem $(11 \times 6) \times 3^2 \div 3 =$, the first step would be to do the parentheses and multiply the 11 by 6 to obtain a product of 66. The second step would be to square the 3, which means 3×3 for a product of 9. The third step would be to multiply the 66×9 for a product of 594. The final step would be to divide the 594 by 3 to obtain the answer of 198.

- *Add or subtract from left to right.* For example, in the problem $(15 + 7) - (8 + 3) + 34 =$, the first steps would be to complete the parentheses: $15 + 7 = 22$ and $8 + 3 = 11$. The problem now reads $22 - 11 + 34 =$. Subtract 11 from 22 to obtain a difference of 11. Then add $11 + 34$ to obtain the answer of 45.

PRACTICAL PROBLEMS

1. Solve the following problems involving combined operations.

    a. $(7 + 9) \times 6 =$ _____

    b. $2 \times (22 + 34) \div 8 =$ _____

    c. $25 \times (8 + 5) - 16 =$ _____

    d. $(154 - 72) \times 43 + (108 - 96)^2 =$ _____

    e. $5^3 \div 25 + (154 - 39) =$ _____

    f. $5,496 - 553 + (6 \times 55) - 7^2 =$ _____

2. A recreational therapist (TR) at a long-term care facility buys 2 bingo games
    at $27 each, 12 puzzles at $5 each, 14 jars of paint at $7 each, 20 paint
    brushes at $2 each, and 24 packages of construction paper at $7 each. How
    much did he spend? _____

3. A licensed practical nurse (LPN) is calculating his patient's oral intake. If the
    patient had 3 large glasses of water containing 240 cubic centimeters (cc)
    each, 2 bowls of broth at 120 cc each, 3 jars of jello at 100 cc each, and 4
    cups of tea at 180 cc each, what amount should be recorded for oral intake
    on the patient's Intake and Output (I & O) record? _____

4. Due to a shortage of workers, a radiologic technologist (RT) is working
    overtime. She gets overtime pay for any hours over eight hours per day. How
    many hours of overtime did she work in one week? _____

DAY OF WEEK	HOURS WORKED
Sunday	0
Monday	13
Tuesday	10
Wednesday	6
Thursday	12
Friday	14
Saturday	11
TOTAL	66

5. A surgical technician (ST) is ordering instruments for the operating room and needs 12 hemostats. One supplier is offering a dozen hemostats for $204, while another supplier charges $16 each for hemostats. If the hemostats are of equal quality, what is the better buy?   _____

6. A phlebotomist does venipunctures to obtain blood samples from patients. One morning he fills 6 vacuum tubes with 12 cubic centimeters (cc) of blood, 3 vacuum tubes with 8 cc of blood, 12 vacuum tubes with 15 cc of blood, and 5 vacuum tubes with 10 cc of blood. How many cc of blood did he obtain from all of his patients?   _____

7. A dental laboratory assistant (DLT) has a 3-pound can of alginate to make impressions. If she uses 2 ounces (oz) of alginate for each impression she makes, how many oz of alginate are left in the can after she makes 11 impressions? (*Hint:* There are 16 oz in one pound.)   _____

8. A worker at a weight loss clinic calculates the number of calories her patients should eat per day. She multiplies the patient's ideal weight by 15 calories if the patient is active and by 20 calories if the patient is very active. She then determines the patient's age and subtracts the number of calories shown on the chart from this daily total of calories to obtain the final correct amount of calories per day.

AGE IN YEARS	CALORIES TO SUBTRACT
25 to 34	0
35 to 44	100
45 to 54	200
55 to 64	300
65 and above	400

a. Mr. Biaski is a very active 47-year-old who should weigh 168 pounds. How many calories should he eat each day?   _____

b. Mrs. Linderman is an active 39-year-old who should weigh 142 pounds. How many calories should she eat each day?   _____

9. An emergency medical technician (EMT) is giving a heart attack victim cardiopulmonary resuscitation (CPR). He gives 2 breaths and 15 compressions in a 15-second period.

    a. How many breaths does he give in 1 minute?   _____

    b. How many chest compressions does he give in 1 minute?   _____

10. A certified biomedical equipment technician (CBET) earns $22 per hour. She is paid double for any hours over 40 hours per week. If she works 49 hours in one week, what is her gross pay?   _____

11. A medical laboratory technologist (MT) is counting leukocytes or white blood cells (WBC). She counts 4 areas on the hemacytometer counting chamber, adds the 4 numbers together, and then multiplies by 50 to obtain the correct leukocyte count. If the counts are 32, 29, 28, and 33, what is the total leukocyte count?   _____

12. A pharmacist is doing an inventory on medications in stock. She finds the following bottles of Synthroid® on the shelf.

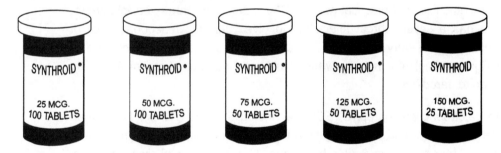

    a. How many tablets of Synthroid® does she have in stock?   _____

    b. How many micrograms (mcg) of Synthroid® does she have in stock?   _____

13. A pediatric assistant is helping a new mother calculate how much formula to buy for her infant. The infant drinks 6 ounces (oz) of formula every four hours (q4h) day and night. The formula is in 1-quart (qt) cans. How many cans will the mother need for 8 days? (*Hint:* 1 qt equals 32 oz.)   _____

14. A certified laboratory technician (CLT) is staining blood film slides with Wright's stain. The Wright's stain bottle contains 120 milliliters (ml). He uses 12 ml of the Wright's stain for each slide and stains 6 slides.

   a. How many ml are left in the bottle after he stains the 6 slides?   _____

   b. How many additional slides can be stained with the Wright's stain?   _____

15. A billing clerk at the hospital is calculating a patient's room charges. The patient spent 3 days in the coronary care unit (CCU), 5 days in the step-down unit, and 7 days in a semiprivate room. What was the total room charge?   _____

TYPE ROOM	DAILY COST
Coronary Care Unit	$1,942
Step-Down Unit	$1,285
Private Room	$896
Semiprivate Room	$747

16. A pediatric licensed practical nurse (LPN) is caring for three-year-old Jared, who has a severe throat infection. He gives Jared 2 teaspoons (tsp) of Ampicillin q6h (every six hours) for three days. If each teaspoon contains 125 milligrams (mg) of Ampicillin, what is the total number of mg of Ampicillin given to Jared?   _____

17. An electroencephalographic (EEG) technologist earns $11 per hour when she works days and $13 per hour when she works nights. One month she works 6 four-hour days, 3 eight-hour days, 3 ten-hour days, 5 six-hour nights, and 4 eight-hour nights. What is her gross pay for the month?   _____

18. A dental lab technician (DLT) has a budget of $2,650 to order supplies for the dental laboratory where he is employed. After he places the order shown, how much of his budget does he have left to spend? _____

QUANTITY	UNITS	ITEM	COST PER ITEM	TOTAL COST
11	Cans	Alginate	$9 per can	
75	Pounds	Lab Plaster	$2 per pound	
50	Pounds	Stone	$3 per pound	
2	Boxes	Custom Tray Mix	$53 per box	
15	Trays	Impression Trays	$8 per tray	
4	Boxes	Baseplate Wax	$11 per box	
			TOTAL	

19. A hematologist must calculate the mean corpuscular hemoglobin concentration (MCHC) of a patient. She uses the formula:

$$MCHC = hemoglobin\ (g/dl) \div hematocrit\ (\%) \times 100$$

A blood test shows that the patient has a hemoglobin of 12 grams per deciliter (gm/dl) and a hematocrit of 48%. What is the patient's MCHC? _____

20. A registered veterinary technician (VTR) is stocking the supply cabinet with flea killing preparations. He stocks 2 cases of spray containing 24 cans per case, 3 cases of shampoo with 12 bottles per case, 4 boxes of foam with 10 cans per case, and 4 cases of powder with 8 boxes per case. Three days later, he calculates that 15 cans of spray, 13 bottles of shampoo, 5 cans of foam, and 11 boxes of powder have been sold to pet owners. How many total items of flea killing preparations are left in the cabinet? _____

21. A health occupations student studies a chart on cancer incidence and deaths to obtain information for a research paper.

LEADING SITES OF CANCER INCIDENCE AND DEATH—2003 ESTIMATES

CANCER INCIDENCE BY SITE AND SEX		CANCER DEATHS BY SITE AND SEX	
MALE	FEMALE	MALE	FEMALE
Prostate 220,900	Breast 211,300	Lung/Bronchus 88,400	Lung/Bronchus 68,800
Lung/Bronchus 91,800	Lung/Bronchus 80,100	Prostate 28,900	Breast 39,800
Colon/Rectum 72,800	Colon/Rectum 74,700	Colon/Rectum 28,300	Colon/Rectum 28,800
Urinary Bladder 42,200	Uterus 40,100	Pancreas 14,700	Pancreas 15,300
Melanoma Skin 29,900	Ovary 25,400	Lymphoma 12,200	Ovary 14,300
Lymphoma 28,300	Lymphoma 25,100	Leukemia 12,100	Lymphoma 11,200
Kidney 19,500	Melanoma Skin 24,300	Esophagus 9,900	Leukemia 9,800
Oral Cavity 18,200	Thyroid 16,300	Liver 9,200	Uterus 6,800
Leukemia 17,900	Pancreas 15,800	Urinary Bladder 8,600	Brain 5,800
Pancreas 14,900	Urinary Bladder 15,200	Kidney 7,400	Multiple Myeloma 5,500
All Sites 675,300	All Sites 658,800	All Sites 285,900	All Sites 270,600

(Courtesy of the American Cancer Society)

a. How many men and women will live after getting lung, colon, or rectal cancer? _____

b. How many men will live after getting cancer of the prostate, urinary bladder, or kidney? _____

c. How many women will live after getting cancer of the breast, ovary, or uterus? _____

d. What cancer site is most likely to cause death in both men and women? _____

Common Fractions

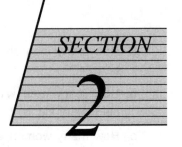

Unit 6 ADDITION OF COMMON FRACTIONS

BASIC PRINCIPLES OF ADDITION OF COMMON FRACTIONS

A common fraction is a quantity that is smaller than a whole number. An example is ¾. This means a whole number has been divided into four parts and the quantity equals three of the four parts. Study the following figure. In this figure, the whole circle is divided into 4 parts. 3 out of the 4 parts of the circle are shaded. The fraction ¾ represents this fact.

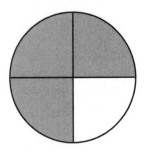

The number above the line in a common fraction is called the *numerator* and the number below the line is called the *denominator*.

Example: 3 = Numerator
⎯
4 = Denominator

Addition When Denominators Are the Same:

When common fractions are added, the denominator of each fraction must be the same. When the denominators are all the same, only the numerators are added. The sum obtained is then placed over the common denominator.

Example: $\frac{1}{12} + \frac{5}{12} + \frac{3}{12}$

$$\frac{1}{12} \qquad 1$$

$$\frac{5}{12} \qquad 5$$

$$+\frac{3}{12} \qquad +\ 3$$

$$\overline{9} \ = \ \frac{9}{12}$$

Addition When Denominators Are Different:

If the denominators are not the same, a *lowest common denominator* must be found. A lowest common denominator is the smallest number that all of the denominators can be divided into evenly. For the numbers $\frac{2}{3}$, $\frac{1}{2}$, and $\frac{1}{4}$, the lowest common denominator would be 12. This is the first number that can be divided evenly by 3, 2, and 4. After the lowest common denominator has been found, each fraction must be converted to a fraction with the lowest common denominator. To do this, divide the denominator of the fraction to be changed into the lowest common denominator to obtain a quotient. Multiply the numerator of the fraction to be changed by this quotient and place this product over the common denominator. Then add the numerators and place this sum over the common denominator to obtain the answer.

Example:

$\frac{2}{3}$	$(12 \div 3 = 4)$	$(2 \times 4 = 8)$ $(3 \times 4 = 12)$	$\frac{8}{12}$
$\frac{1}{2}$	$(12 \div 2 = 6)$	$(1 \times 6 = 6)$ $(2 \times 6 = 12)$	$\frac{6}{12}$
$+\frac{1}{4}$	$(12 \div 4 = 3)$	$(1 \times 3 = 3)$ $(4 \times 3 = 12)$	$+\dfrac{3}{12}$
			$\dfrac{17}{12}$

Reducing a Fraction to Its Lowest Terms:

A fraction must also be reduced to its lowest terms. In the answers for the previous examples, both $^9/_{12}$ and $^{17}/_{12}$ are not in lowest terms. In $^9/_{12}$, both the 9 and the 12 can be divided by 3. To reduce the fraction, divide both the numerator and denominator by the same number to obtain the correct answer. In this case, it is $^3/_4$.

Example:

$$\frac{9}{12} \quad \begin{matrix}(9 \div 3 = 3) \\ (12 \div 3 = 4)\end{matrix} \quad = \quad \frac{3}{4}$$

The fraction $^{17}/_{12}$ represents a quantity greater than the denominator of 12. To reduce this fraction, divide the 17 by 12. The quotient will have a whole number of 1 with a remainder of 5. The remainder is placed over the denominator of the original fraction and a mixed number is the answer. A *mixed number* is a mixture of a whole number and a fraction.

Example:

$$\frac{17}{12} \qquad 17 \div 12 = 1 \text{ with R } 5 \qquad \text{Answer: } 1\ ^5/_{12}$$

Addition of Mixed Numbers:

To add mixed numbers, line up the numbers in a column. Add the whole numbers together first. Then make sure the fractions all have a common denominator or convert them to fractions with a common denominator. Add the numerators together, write the sum obtained over the common denominator, and reduce the fraction as necessary. If a whole number is obtained while reducing the fraction, add it to the sum of the whole numbers. Then write the sum of the whole numbers and the fraction as the answer.

Example: $1^1/_2 + 3^3/_4$

$$
\begin{array}{llll}
1 & \dfrac{1}{2} & (4 \div 2 = 2) & \begin{matrix}(1 \times 2 = 2)\\(2 \times 2 = 4)\end{matrix} & 1\ \dfrac{2}{4}\\[2ex]
\underline{+\ 3} & \underline{\dfrac{3}{4}} & & & \underline{+\ 3\ \dfrac{3}{4}}\\[2ex]
4 & & & & \dfrac{5}{4} \quad = \quad 1\dfrac{1}{4}
\end{array}
$$

$$
\begin{array}{ll}
4 & \\
\underline{+\ 1} & \underline{\dfrac{1}{4}}\\[2ex]
5 & \dfrac{1}{4} \qquad \text{Answer: } 5^1/_4
\end{array}
$$

PRACTICAL PROBLEMS

1. Add the following fractions:

    a. $\frac{3}{8} + \frac{5}{8} + \frac{1}{8}$ _____

    b. $\frac{1}{8} + \frac{3}{4} + \frac{1}{2}$ _____

    c. $2\frac{3}{4} + 1\frac{3}{4}$ _____

    d. $3\frac{5}{8} + 20\frac{3}{5}$ _____

    e. $7\frac{3}{10} + 18\frac{4}{5} + 26\frac{5}{8} + 14\frac{3}{4}$ _____

    f. $8\frac{5}{12} + 106\frac{3}{4} + 77\frac{5}{6} + 23\frac{7}{10}$ _____

2. A licensed practical nurse (LPN) gives a patient $\frac{1}{4}$ ounce (oz) of cough medicine at 6 PM and $\frac{3}{4}$ oz of cough medicine at 10 PM. How much cough medicine does she give? _____

3. A pediatric assistant is calculating the growth of an infant. The baby grew $\frac{5}{8}$ inch (") during the first month of life, $\frac{1}{4}$" the second month, and $\frac{5}{16}$" the third month. How much did the infant grow? _____

4. A surgical nurse in an outpatient surgical clinic works $1\frac{1}{4}$ hours in preoperative care (before surgery), $2\frac{1}{2}$ hours in the operating room, and $3\frac{3}{4}$ hours in the recovery room. How many hours does she work each day? _____

5. An occupational therapist (OT) is keeping a record on the physical activity of a cardiac patient. He records how far the patient walks each day. How many miles did the patient walk for the week? _____

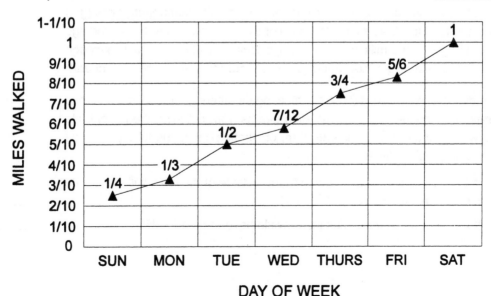

6. An allergist gives a patient a series of injections to desensitize the patient for allergies. She administers ¼ milliliter (ml) of the solution the first week, ½ ml the second week, ¾ ml the third week, 1 ml the fourth week, and 1¼ ml the fifth week. How many milliliters did the patient receive in the five-week period?

    _____

7. A patient care technician (PCT) in a newborn nursery weighs a set of quadruplets when they are born. The infants weigh 3¼ pounds (lb), 2⅝ lb, 2½ lb, and 3⅜ lb. What is the total weight for all four infants?

    _____

8. A medical laboratory technician (MLT) uses ½ ounce (oz), ¼ oz, and ⅜ oz of solution to perform 3 urinary sedimentation tests. How much total solution does she use?

    _____

9. A dental assistant (DA) is developing dental X rays. He follows the time chart recommended for the speed film he is using. What is the total time required to complete the developing process?

    _____

DEVELOPING PROCESS	TIME REQUIRED
Developer	2 ½ minutes
Rinse	½ minute
Fix Solution	3 ¼ minutes
Final Wash	20 minutes

10. A dietetic technician (DT) helps a patient calculate the number of grams (gm) of saturated fat. If the patient ate 1 slice of bacon with 1¼ gm, 1 poached egg with 1½ gm, 1 cup milk with 2¾ gm, 1 biscuit with 1¼ gm, and 1 teaspoon margarine with ½ gm, how many grams of saturated fat did the patient eat?

    _____

11. A radiologic technologist (RT) is evaluating the filtering effect of aluminum in preventing the lower energy radiation beams from reaching the patient. He knows that there is ½ millimeter (mm) of filtration inside the tube to provide inherent or built-in filtration.

    a. If 1½ mm of aluminum is added to the outside of the tube, will this create the ideal beam filtration of 2½ mm?

    _____

    b. If not, how much more aluminum would have to be added?

    _____

12. A paramedic maintains a time card for hours she works on the rescue squad. How many hours did she work per week?   _____

DAY OF WEEK	HOURS WORKED
Sunday	$6\frac{1}{2}$
Monday	$8\frac{1}{4}$
Tuesday	0
Wednesday	$7\frac{3}{4}$
Thursday	$8\frac{1}{12}$
Friday	$8\frac{5}{12}$
Saturday	0
TOTAL	

13. A hospice nurse administers $\frac{1}{6}$ grain (gr) of morphine sulfate to a cancer patient. Four hours later she gives the patient $\frac{1}{8}$ gr. What is the total dose of morphine given to the patient?   _____

14. A student receives her college schedule for her first semester of study in a pharmacy technician program.

Course	Semester Hours
Communications	2
Orientation	$\frac{1}{4}$
Study Skills	$\frac{1}{4}$
Anatomy and Physiology	$2\frac{1}{2}$
Anatomy and Physiology Lab	$1\frac{1}{2}$
Advanced Algebra	$2\frac{1}{4}$
Physical Education	$\frac{1}{2}$

What is the total number of semester hours?   _____

15. A dental assistant (DA) calculates the number of ounces of disinfectant required to clean the dental operatory between patients. He uses $1\frac{3}{8}$ ounces (oz) of disinfectant for the dental chair, $\frac{1}{6}$ oz for the low-speed handpiece, $\frac{1}{4}$ oz for the high-speed handpiece, $\frac{5}{12}$ oz for the light, and $\frac{1}{2}$ oz for the dental cart. What is the total amount of disinfectant used? _____

16. An intensive care unit nurse graphs the amount of Coumadin® given to a stroke patient in a six-day period.

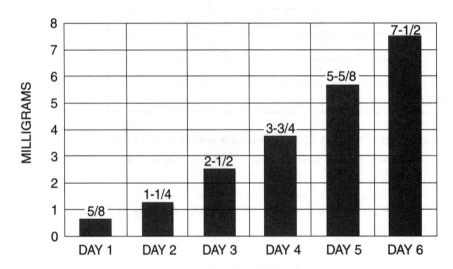

COUMADIN® DOSAGE

a. How many milligrams (mg) of Coumadin® did the patient receive in the first three days? _____

b. How many mg did the patient receive during the six days? _____

c. How many additional mg did the patient receive on the last day as compared to the first day dose? _____

Unit 7 *SUBTRACTION OF COMMON FRACTIONS*

BASIC PRINCIPLES OF SUBTRACTION OF COMMON FRACTIONS

Subtraction of common fractions follows the same principles as addition of common fractions. If the denominators are the same, the numerators are subtracted and the difference is put over the common denominator. If the denominators are not the same, the fractions must be converted to fractions with a lowest common denominator before the numerators can be subtracted. The fractional difference must then be reduced to lowest terms.

Example: $\frac{9}{16} - \frac{1}{4}$

$$\frac{9}{16} \qquad\qquad\qquad\qquad\qquad\qquad\qquad\qquad\qquad \frac{9}{16}$$

$$-\ \frac{1}{4} \qquad (16 \div 4 = 4) \qquad (1 \times 4 = 4) \qquad\qquad -\ \frac{4}{16}$$

$$\qquad\qquad\qquad\qquad\qquad\qquad\qquad (4 \times 4 = 16) \qquad\qquad \frac{5}{16}$$

When mixed numbers are subtracted, the fractional part of each mixed number must first be converted to the lowest common denominator. If the numerator of the fraction in the subtrahend (number to be subtracted) is larger than the numerator of the fraction in the minuend (number from which it is to be subtracted), one unit must be borrowed from the whole number in the minuend. The mixed number $5\frac{3}{4}$ is equal to $4 + \frac{4}{4} + \frac{3}{4}$. The $\frac{4}{4}$ represents the one unit borrowed from the whole number which in turn has become 4 instead of 5. When the fractional parts are added, the number becomes $4\frac{7}{4}$. Subtraction then proceeds by subtracting the numerators of the fractional parts and the whole numbers.

Example: 6¼ − 3⅔

$$6 \quad \frac{1}{4} \qquad (12 \div 4 = 3) \qquad (1 \times 3 = 3) \qquad 6 \quad \frac{3}{12} \; (5 = {}^{12}\!/_{12} + {}^{3}\!/_{12})$$

$$\qquad\qquad\qquad\qquad\qquad (4 \times 3 = 12)$$

$$- \quad 3\frac{2}{3} \qquad (12 \div 3 = 4) \qquad (2 \times 4 = 8) \qquad - \; 3 \quad \frac{8}{12}$$

$$\qquad\qquad\qquad\qquad\qquad (3 \times 4 = 12)$$

$$5 \quad \frac{15}{12}$$

$$- \qquad 3 \quad \frac{8}{12}$$

$$2 \quad \frac{7}{12}$$

PRACTICAL PROBLEMS

1. Subtract the following fractions:

    a. $^{15}\!/_{16} - ^{3}\!/_{8}$ _____

    b. $9^{3}\!/_{4} - 6^{5}\!/_{6}$ _____

    c. $5 - ^{7}\!/_{16}$ _____

    d. $46^{3}\!/_{4} - 37^{1}\!/_{3}$ _____

    e. $146^{3}\!/_{5} - 97^{7}\!/_{8}$ _____

    f. $211^{15}\!/_{16} - 189^{57}\!/_{64}$ _____

2. An ophthalmic assistant gets overtime pay for all hours over 40 hours per week. If he works $48^{3}\!/_{4}$ hours, how many hours of overtime does he work? _____

3. A medical laboratory technologist (MT) notes that a patient's hemoglobin (hgb) level was $10^{1}\!/_{2}$ grams (gm) after surgery. The patient then received two pints of blood and the hgb level was 15 gm. What was the increase in the hemoglobin level after the patient received the blood? _____

4. A surgical technician (ST) must make sure that 20 pints (pt) of normal saline (NS) solution are in stock. At the end of one day, he has $11^{2}\!/_{3}$ pt. How many pints of NS solution were used during the day? _____

5. A diet consultant graphs the one-month weight loss for a patient who weighed 278¾ pounds. How much did the patient weigh after 4 weeks of dieting? _____

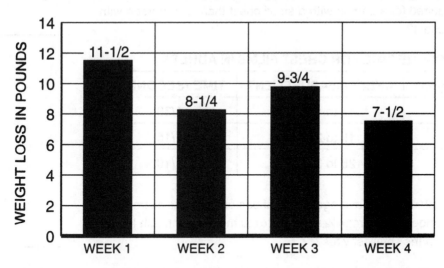

6. A pediatric nurse measures one-year-old Nicky and finds that he is 37¼ inches (") tall. At birth, Nicky was 18¾" tall. How much did Nicky grow in one year? _____

7. A medical secretary is designing an information sheet on postoperative care. If she has 1½-inch margins at the top and bottom of an 11-inch sheet of paper, how much room does she have left for the written information? _____

8. A dietetic assistant prepares 36 ounces (oz) of formula for the infants in the pediatric nursery. If the infants drink 3½ oz, 4¼ oz, 3¾ oz, 4½ oz, and 3¼ oz, how much formula is left? _____

9. A radiologic technologist (RT) studies the following chart on time required to take a chest X ray based on the size of a person's chest. How much less time in seconds is required for a person with a small chest than for a person with the largest size chest?   _____

EXPOSURE TIME FOR CHEST FILMS IN ADULTS

MILLIAMPS (mA)	CHEST MEASUREMENT	TIME (SECONDS)
300	15 to 18 cm	1/30
300	19 to 22 cm	1/15
300	25 to 32 cm	1/10

10. A microbiologist notes that the average length of bacteria is $1/1000$ micrometer (mcm). Viruses range in size from $1/2,5000$ to $1/50,000$ mcm. How much longer is a bacterium than the smallest virus?   _____

11. A dental hygienist (DH) is in charge of the construction of a new dental X-ray unit. She knows the walls must be at least $2\frac{5}{8}$ inches (") thick if gypsum sheet rock is used or $1/16$" thick if sheets of lead are embedded in the wall to prevent the passage of X-radiation. What is the difference in the thickness of the walls?   _____

12. A physician's assistant (PA) measures two twin girls, Karen and Kathy. Karen has grown $3/4$ inch (") and Kathy has grown $7/16$".

    a. Which twin has grown the most?   _____

    b. How much taller has she grown?   _____

13. An inspector for the United States Environmental Protection Agency (EPA) informs the owners of a company that they must not allow workers into one warehouse because the radioactive radon gas level in the building measures 15¾ picocuries (a measurement of radiation) per liter (l) of air. The average household level is 1¼ picocuries.

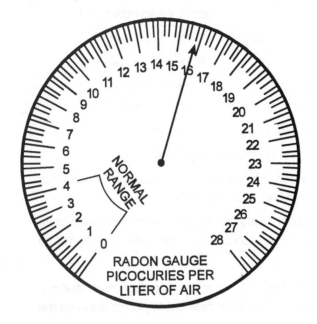

a. How much higher is the radon level in the warehouse than the highest normal radon level?   _____

b. How much higher is the radon level in the warehouse than the average household level?   _____

14. A statistician for the Centers for Disease Control and Prevention (CDC) is studying the effectiveness of the Hepatitis B vaccine. By checking antibody levels in the blood five years after administration of the vaccine, he finds that ⅕ of the people under 30 years of age, ¼ of the people 30 to 40 years of age, and ⅓ of the people over 40 years of age are not protected.

a. What age group has the best protection after 5 years?   _____

b. What greater fraction of those people over 40 compared to people under 30 are not protected?   _____

15. A student enrolled in a radiology program evaluates information about exposure to environmental or naturally occurring background radiation. She notes that the following exposures are present in milliSieverts (mSv), a measure of radiation exposure:

AREA	LEVEL OF EXPOSURE
Eastern and Central United States	$\frac{1}{3}$ to $\frac{3}{4}$ mSv/year
Atlantic and Gulf Coastal Plain	$\frac{3}{4}$ to $1\frac{1}{2}$ mSv/year
Colorado Plateau Area	$\frac{3}{20}$ to $\frac{1}{3}$ mSv/year

a. What area has the highest level of radiation exposure?   _____

b. What area has the lowest level of radiation exposure?   _____

c. What is the difference between the highest level shown in the statistics and the lowest level of radiation exposure in mSv?   _____

d. Why do you think individuals living at higher elevations have more exposure to radiation? (*Hint:* The atmosphere helps filter radiation from the sun.)   _____

16. A recreational therapist (TR) is evaluating how long a person must perform certain activities to exercise moderately. After researching information on the Internet, she compiles the following chart:

TYPE ACTIVITY	TIME REQUIRED (HOURS)
Playing Volleyball	3/4
Gardening or Weeding Flower Beds	2/3
Wheeling Self in Wheelchair	5/6
Riding a Bicycle	1/2
Swimming Laps in a Pool	25/60
Walking Up and Down Stairs	1/4

a. What activity requires the longest period of time to exercise moderately?   _____

b. How much longer must a person garden instead of swimming laps in a pool?   _____

c. How much longer must a person wheel himself or herself in a wheelchair instead of walking up and down stairs?   _____

Unit 8 MULTIPLICATION OF COMMON FRACTIONS

BASIC PRINCIPLES OF MULTIPLICATION OF COMMON FRACTIONS

To multiply common fractions, multiply the numerators, then multiply the denominators, and, if necessary, reduce the answer to the lowest terms. It is not necessary to have the same denominators for multiplication.

Example: $\frac{2}{3} \times \frac{5}{8}$

$$\frac{2}{3} \quad \times \quad \frac{5}{8} \quad = \quad \frac{2 \times 5 =}{3 \times 8 =} \quad \frac{10}{24} \quad \begin{matrix} (10 \div 2 = 5) \\ (24 \div 2 = 12) \end{matrix} \quad \begin{matrix} = \\ = \end{matrix} \quad \frac{5}{12}$$

If a number in the numerator and a number in the denominator can both be divided by the same number, smaller numbers can be obtained before multiplication occurs.

Example: $\frac{3}{4} \times \frac{5}{12}$

$$\frac{3}{4} \quad \times \quad \frac{5}{12} \quad = \quad \frac{1\cancel{3}}{4} \quad (3 \div 3 = 1) \quad \times \quad \frac{5}{4\,\cancel{12}} \quad (12 \div 3 = 4) \quad = \frac{5}{16}$$

To multiply mixed numbers, convert the mixed number to an improper fraction. An improper fraction is a fraction greater than a whole number. To do this, multiply the whole number by the denominator and add the product to the numerator. Put this sum over the original denominator.

Example: $7\frac{2}{3} = \frac{(7 \times 3 = 21 + 2 = 23)}{3} = \frac{23}{3}$

To multiply a whole number by a fraction, put the whole number over a denominator of 1.

Example: $4 \times 6\frac{1}{2}$

$$\frac{4}{1} \quad \times \quad \frac{(6 \times 2 = 12 + 1 = 13)}{2} \quad \frac{13}{2}$$

$$\frac{4}{1} \quad \times \quad \frac{13}{2} \quad = \quad \frac{2\cancel{4}}{1} \quad \times \quad \frac{13}{1\cancel{2}} \quad = \quad \frac{26}{1} \quad = \quad 26$$

PRACTICAL PROBLEMS

1. Multiply the following fractions:

   a. $\frac{3}{4} \times \frac{3}{8}$ _____

   b. $\frac{7}{12} \times \frac{8}{21}$ _____

   c. $5 \times 9\frac{2}{3}$ _____

   d. $12\frac{2}{5} \times 5\frac{5}{8}$ _____

   e. $34\frac{2}{3} \times 41\frac{5}{6}$ _____

   f. $5\frac{7}{10} \times 106\frac{8}{15}$ _____

2. A neonatal nurse (RN) weighs a newborn baby. The baby weighs $6\frac{3}{4}$ pounds (lb). If the infant triples his weight in 1 year, how much should the infant weigh when he is 1 year old? _____

3. A hospital administrator must decrease the staff size by $\frac{1}{12}$ because of budget cuts. If the hospital employs 456 people, how many people must be dismissed? _____

4. A pharmaceutical company technician uses a 240-milliliter (ml) flask of vaccine solution to fill individual vials. If each vial is $\frac{1}{15}$ of the volume of the flask, how many ml of vaccine are in each vial? _____

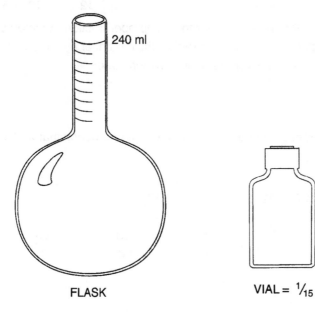

240 ml

FLASK   VIAL = $\frac{1}{15}$

5. A registered nurse (RN) gives a patient ½ tablet of morphine for pain. If one morphine tablet contains ¼ grain (gr), how much morphine does the patient receive? _____

6. A sophomore in high school is considering a career in health care. She learns that approximately 5,328,524 people are employed in health care. If ½ of these people work in hospitals, how many people work in hospitals? _____

7. After developing X rays, the radiologic technician finds that the image is dark and nothing is visible. He knows that the milliampere-seconds (mAs) for the X-ray machine should be reduced to ¼ of what was originally used to correct this problem. If he used 40 mAs to take the X rays, what should he use to correct the problem? _____

8. An electrocardiographic (ECG) technician knows that one small horizontal block on ECG paper represents ¹⁄₂₅ of a second.

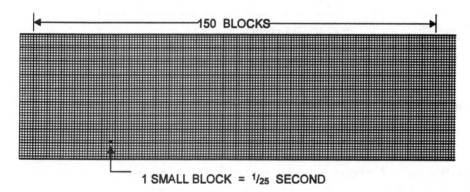

a. How many seconds are represented by 5 small blocks? _____

b. How many seconds are represented by 150 small blocks? _____

9. A licensed practical nurse (LPN) gives a patient 2½ tablets of acetaminophen. If each tablet contains 300 milligrams (mg), how many mg of acetaminophen does the patient receive? _____

10. A home health care assistant prepares 48 ounces (oz) of infant formula. The mixture is ⅓ formula and ⅔ water.

a. How much formula does she use to make 48 oz total? _____

b. How much water does she use to make 48 oz total? _____

11. A student doing a research paper on acquired immune deficiency syndrome (AIDS) learns that $\frac{1}{6}$ of the people with AIDS are in their 20s. Since the latency period between the time of the HIV infection and the onset of AIDS is about 10 years, most of these people were infected as teenagers. If there are 133,758 cases of AIDS, how many were probably infected as teenagers? _____

12. An athletic trainer (AT) is checking a box of cereal to find the content of various nutrients. She knows that $\frac{1}{15}$ of each of the nutrients represents one serving of cereal. How many of each nutrient are in one serving of cereal?

NUTRIENT	AMOUNT	PER SERVING
Cholesterol	0 milligrams (mg)	
Sodium	3,300 mg	
Potassium	375 mg	
Total Carbohydrates	405 grams (gm)	
Dietary Fiber	15 gm	
Sugars	165 gm	
Other Carbohydrates	225 gm	
Protein	30 gm	

13. A surgical nurse (RN) works $7\frac{1}{2}$ hours a day. He spends $\frac{1}{2}$ of the time in the operating room, $\frac{1}{4}$ in the recovery room, $\frac{1}{8}$ in sterile supply, and $\frac{1}{8}$ in medical records.

   a. How many hours does he work in the operating room? _____

   b. How many hours does he work in the recovery room? _____

   c. How many hours does he work in sterile supply and medical records? _____

14. A biomedical equipment technician (BET) is measuring the heat unit capacity of an X-ray tube. She uses the following formula:

    Heat Units (HU) = mA (milliamperes) × Time × kV (kilovoltage)

    If she knows the mA is 200, the time is ⅕ a second, and the kV is 50, what is the capacity in heat units?   _____

15. A radiologist is measuring the amount of radiation exposure a patient receives during a chest X ray. She expresses the exposure in milliampere-seconds (mAs) after multiplying the time of exposure in seconds by the milliamperage (mA) used. If she uses 300 mA for ¹⁄₃₀ of a second to take the X ray, how much exposure does the patient receive?   _____

    Note: Use the following chart to complete problems 16−18.

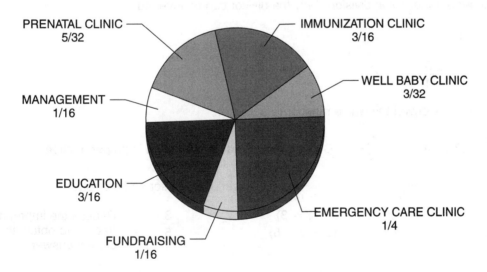

COMMUNITY HEALTH CARE SERVICES
ANNUAL BUDGET $680,288

16. What is the total amount in dollars that Community Health Care Services spends for education?   _____

17. What is the total amount in dollars that Community Health Care Services spends for different clinics?   _____

18. What is the total amount in dollars that Community Health Care Services spends for management and fundraising?   _____

Unit 9 DIVISION OF COMMON FRACTIONS

BASIC PRINCIPLES OF DIVISION OF COMMON FRACTIONS

In order to divide fractions, the divisor must be inverted. To do this, reverse or interchange the numerator and denominator. Then proceed following the same rules used for multiplication of fractions.

Example: $\frac{5}{8} \div \frac{2}{3}$

$$\frac{5}{8} \div \frac{2}{3} = \frac{5}{8} \times \frac{3}{2} = \frac{15}{16}$$

To divide whole numbers, write the number as a fraction. For example, the number 6 is written as $\frac{6}{1}$. To divide mixed numbers, first convert the mixed number to an improper fraction. For example, the number $3\frac{3}{4}$ is the same as $\frac{15}{4}$. Then invert the divisor and follow the rules for multiplication of fractions. Remember that order is important in division. Only the divisor can be inverted.

Example: $6 \div 3\frac{3}{4}$

$$6 \div 3\frac{3}{4} = ?$$

$6 = \frac{6}{1}$ Convert the whole number to a fraction.

$3\frac{3}{4} = (3 \times 4) + 3 = \frac{15}{4}$ Convert the mixed number to an improper fraction.

$\frac{6}{1} \times \frac{4}{15} = \frac{24}{15}$ Invert the devisor and multiply.

$\frac{24}{15} = 1\frac{9}{15}$ $\begin{array}{c}(9 \div 3 = 3)\\(15 \div 3 = 5)\end{array}$ $= 1\frac{3}{5}$ Reduce the improper fraction to obtain the correct answer.

PRACTICAL PROBLEMS

1. Divide the following fractions:

    a. $\frac{7}{8} \div \frac{5}{6}$ _____

    b. $9\frac{1}{2} \div 4\frac{3}{8}$ _____

    c. $7 \div \frac{2}{3}$ _____

    d. $27\frac{1}{2} \div 5\frac{1}{2}$ _____

    e. $\frac{3}{4} \div 60$ _____

    f. $18\frac{3}{4} \div 3\frac{5}{8}$ _____

2. A veterinary assistant worked $42\frac{1}{2}$ hours in a 5-day week. If she worked the same number of hours each day, how many hours did she work per day?   _____

3. A pharmacist has a 9-gram (gm) vial of medication. How many $\frac{2}{3}$-gm doses can be obtained from this vial?   _____

4. A registered nurse (RN) fills a syringe with $1\frac{1}{2}$ cubic centimeters (cc) of normal saline (NS) solution. This is $\frac{1}{20}$ of the amount in the vial of NS. How many cc of NS are in the vial? (*Hint:* Division of fractions can provide a total amount when a part is known. The part is divided by the fraction that it represents to get the total amount. In this case, $\frac{1}{20}$ is the divisor.)   _____

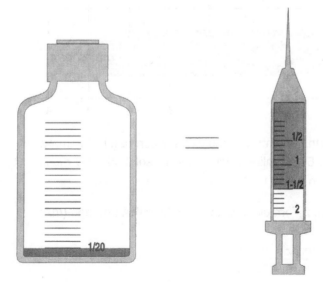

5. A student working on a Bachelor of Science (BS) degree in nursing has completed 68½ semester hours, or ½ of the required hours. How many semester hours does he need for the degree?

    _____

6. A patient is told to take 12½ grains (gr) of aspirin qd (every day). If the aspirin tablets contain 5 gr each, how many tablets must the patient take qd?

    _____

7. Statistics show that about 1 out of 1,000 of all people with hepatitis die each year of fulminant hepatitis, a rapidly fatal form of the disease. If 250 people die of fulminant hepatitis each year, how many cases of hepatitis occur each year? (*Hint:* Write 1 out of 1,000 as the fraction ¹⁄₁,₀₀₀ and use this fraction as the divisor.)

    _____

8. Two surgical technicians (STs) work in the operating room five days each week. In a one-week period, how many times longer does technician 2 work as compared to technician 1?

    _____

HOURS WORKED PER DAY

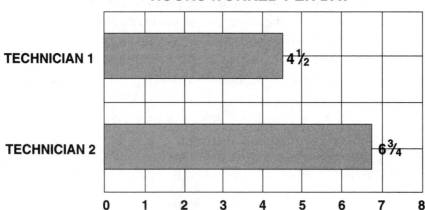

9. A cardiac care nurse notes that an intravenous (IV) solution bag is ⅖ empty. If the patient has absorbed 600 milliliters (ml) of the IV solution, how much solution was in the bag when it was full?

    _____

10. A radiologist uses the following formula to determine the milliAmperage (mA) setting for the X-ray machine:

    $$mA = \frac{\text{milliamp-seconds (mAs)}}{\text{exposure time in seconds}}$$

    If she uses 10 mAs for ¹⁄₂₀ of a second, what should the mA setting be?

    _____

11. A medical records technician notes that 3 out of 8 patients or a total of 7,743 patients admitted to the hospital in a one-year period had heart or lung disease. How many total patients were admitted to the hospital during the year? (*Hint:* Remember to write 3 out of 8 as the fraction ⅜.) _____

12. A licensed practical nurse (LPN) is told to give 5½ milligrams (mg) of Coumadin® to a heart attack patient. If the tablets are 2 mg, how many tablets must he give to the patient? _____

13. A dialysis technician notes that $135 was taken out of her paycheck for federal tax, state tax, city tax, and FICA. This is ³⁄₁₀ of her paycheck.

    a. What is her gross pay per week? _____

    b. What is her gross pay per hour if she works 37½ hours per week? _____

14. A director of a home care service calculates that ¹⁄₁₂ of the budget is spent for supplies and ⅙ for transportation costs. If supplies and transportation costs are $83,595, what is the total budget? _____

15. A patient care technician (PCT) notes that a patient's water pitcher is still ¼ full. If the patient drank 1125 cubic centimeters (cc) of water, how many cc of water does a full pitcher hold? (*Hint:* Note that the 1125 cc of water does not represent ¼ of the pitcher.) _____

16. A radioactive isotope used for radiation treatments has the following half-life (it loses ½ of its radioactivity, measured in milliSieverts (mSv), in a specific period of time). Show your formula and determine the original measurement of radioactivity in mSv. _____

ORIGINAL RADIOACTIVITY   **1ST HALF-LIFE**

2ND HALF-LIFE   **3RD HALF-LIFE**

20 mSv   10 mSv

Unit 10 COMBINED OPERATIONS WITH COMMON FRACTIONS

BASIC PRINCIPLES OF COMBINED OPERATIONS WITH COMMON FRACTIONS

Follow all of the rules for addition, subtraction, multiplication, and division of common fractions to solve the problems in this unit.

PRACTICAL PROBLEMS

1. Perform the operations indicated:

   a. $\frac{1}{2} + \frac{1}{4} + \frac{1}{8} =$ _____

   b. $\dfrac{5 \times \frac{5}{8}}{\frac{1}{2}} + \dfrac{3}{4} =$ _____

   c. $\dfrac{5\frac{1}{2} \times \frac{2}{3}}{\frac{1}{4}} - 4\frac{3}{12}$ _____

   d. $\dfrac{1\frac{3}{8} + \frac{5}{16} + \frac{7}{32}}{\frac{1}{2}} \times \dfrac{5\frac{2}{3}}{2\frac{1}{6}}$ _____

2. An emergency medical technician (EMT) earns $9 per hour and works $8\frac{1}{2}$ hours each day. A paramedic earns $16 per hour and works $7\frac{3}{4}$ hours each day. If they both work 5 days each week, how much more does the paramedic earn for the week? _____

3. A one-month old infant drinks $3\frac{3}{4}$ ounces (oz) of formula q4h (every four hours) except when he sleeps from 10 PM to 6 AM.

   a. How many oz does the infant drink in 1 day? _____

   b. How many oz does the infant drink in 1 week? _____

4. A patient is taking $2\frac{1}{2}$ milligrams (mg) of Valium® tid (three times a day). If each Valium® tablet contains 5 mg, how many tablets does the patient take qd (every day)? _____

5. A geriatric assistant (GA) must calculate the total cubic centimeters (cc) of oral intake for a resident's Intake and Output (I & O) record. The patient drank 1⅔ cups of coffee, ¾ of a glass of juice, 1⅚ glasses of water, ¾ of a small bowl of jello (counted as a liquid oral intake), and ½ of a large bowl of soup. What is the resident's total oral intake?   _____

CONTAINER	CONTENTS
Juice Glass	120 cc
Water Glass	180 cc
Large Glass	240 cc
Small Bowl	100 cc
Large Bowl	200 cc
Cup	180 cc
Coffee Pot	360 cc

6. A staining solution bottle in a medical laboratory contains 30 ounces (oz). A blood staining test requires ¾ oz of solution. A tissue staining test requires ½ oz of solution. If 4 blood tests and 5 tissue tests are performed, how many oz of solution are left in the bottle?   _____

7. A dentist has to buy a new air compressor to run the handpieces on the dental unit. She knows the high-speed handpiece requires ⅜ horsepower (HP), the low-speed handpiece requires ½ HP, and the air-water syringe requires 3⁄16 HP.

   a. Would a 1-HP air compressor run all three handpieces at the same time?   _____

   b. Why or why not?   _____

8. A pharmacist weighs a 500-milligram (mg) capsule of Ampicillin and finds that it weighs 3⁄20 of an ounce. How much would 50 capsules containing 250 mg weigh?   _____

9.   A premature infant is weighed daily to calculate weight gain or loss.

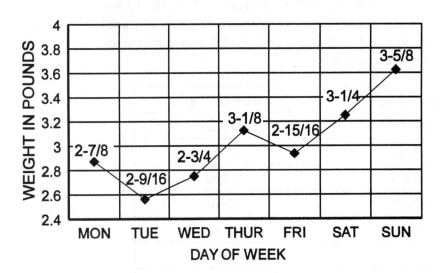

a. How many pounds (lb) did the premature infant lose during the week?   _____

b. How many lb did the premature infant gain during the week?   _____

c. What was the difference in weight between the first day and the last day?   _____

10.   A hospital employs 256 people.

a. If $\frac{5}{8}$ of the employees are nurses, how many nurses does the hospital employ?   _____

b. If $\frac{1}{8}$ of the employees work in radiology, $\frac{1}{16}$ in respiratory therapy, and $\frac{3}{16}$ in the medical laboratory, what is the total number of people working in these areas?   _____

11.   An ulcer patient is taking Mylanta® from a 36-ounce (oz) bottle. If he takes $\frac{3}{4}$ oz qoh (every other hour) beginning at 6 AM and ending with a final dose at 10 PM, how many days would a bottle last?   _____

12. A medical secretary has a 4-drawer file cabinet. One drawer is ⅘ full, one drawer is ½ full, one drawer is ⅔ full, and 1 drawer is ¾ full. Can the contents be combined into 3 drawers? Explain why or why not.   _____

13. An oncologist examines a chart on the cases of cancer by type in his state.

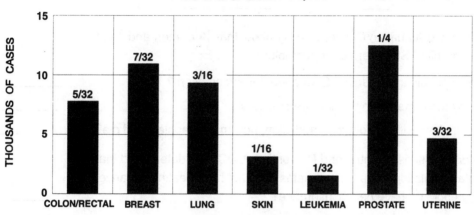

CANCER CASES BY TYPE
TOTAL CASES - 48,096

TYPE OF CANCER

a. What fraction represents the number of cases of colon/rectal and lung cancer?   _____

b. How many people have colon/rectal and lung cancer?   _____

c. How many more cases of prostate cancer are there than cancers of the uterus?   _____

d. How many more women have either breast or uterine cancer than men have prostate cancer?   _____

14. A physical therapist assistant works 42½ hours per week for $12 per hour. His gross pay is reduced by ⅕ for federal tax, ³⁄₅₀ for state tax, and ¹⁄₁₀₀ for local tax. How much money does he receive for two weeks of work after these deductions are taken out?   _____

Note: Use the following figures (rounded to hundred thousands) from the United States Census Bureau to answer questions 15–17.

POPULATION	NUMBER
Males	138,100,000
Females	143,400,000
TOTAL POPULATION	281,000,000

15. Statistics from the American Cancer Society show that ¼ of men and ⅕ of women in the United States are current smokers.

    a. How many people in the United States are current smokers?   _____

    b. How many more men than woman are smokers?   _____

    c. If ⁹⁄₂₀ of smokers will die from their addiction, how many people could die?   _____

16. The Centers for Disease Control and Prevention (CDC) has determined that ⅖ of the total population in the United States does not have health insurance. How many people do have health insurance?   _____

17. The CDC also estimates that ⁶⁄₂₅ of the population in the United States is obese or overweight. How many people are not overweight?   _____

18. Statistics show that since the advent of the Hepatitis B vaccine, the annual number of people infected with Hepatitis B has dropped from 240,000 to 78,200. The statistics for this group of individuals are shown in the following chart:

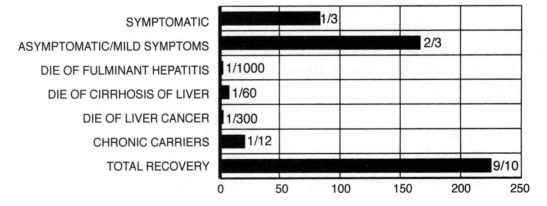

HEPATITIS CASES
THOUSANDS

a. How many people die of fulminant hepatitis, cirrhosis, or cancer of the liver?   _____

b. How many people recover completely from Hepatitis B or become carriers (individuals who spread the disease to others)?   _____

c. If people die of hepatitis only after having symptoms of the disease, how many with symptoms will die of the disease?   _____

d. How many fewer individuals become carriers of Hepatitis B than when the number of cases was 240,000 per year?   _____

19. A hemacytometer counting chamber is used to count both erythrocytes (red blood cells or RBCs) and leukocytes (white blood cells or WBCs). The areas for counting each type of cell are shown on the diagram.

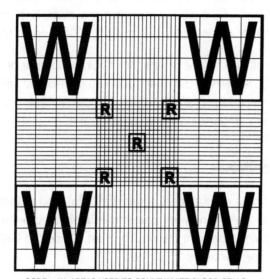

CODE: W=AREAS USED TO COUNT WHITE BLOOD CELLS
R=AREAS USED TO COUNT RED BLOOD CELLS

a. What fractional part of the entire slide is used for counting WBCs?   _____

b. What fractional part of the entire slide is used for counting RBCs?   _____

Decimal Fractions

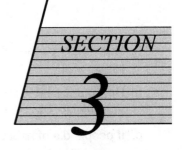

Unit 11 ADDITION OF DECIMAL FRACTIONS

BASIC PRINCIPLES OF ADDITION OF DECIMAL FRACTIONS

Decimals are fractions with denominators of 10 or multiples of 10. They are similar to common fractions because they represent a part of a whole unit. However, a decimal fraction is written as a whole number with a period in front of it. Each place after the period represents a multiple of 10. The fraction $^4\!/_{10}$ represents the decimal 0.4, $^4\!/_{100}$ is 0.04, $^4\!/_{1,000}$ is 0.004, $^4\!/_{10,000}$ is 0.0004, and so forth.

It is important to remember that zeros placed before or after the decimal number do not alter or change the number. For example, .4 can also be written as 0.4, 0.40, or 0.400. In medical fields, a zero is usually placed before a decimal point to avoid misreading a number as a whole number. For example, .4 would be written as 0.4 to prevent reading the number as a whole number of 4.

Components of a Decimal Fraction:

Decimal fractions have three parts: a whole number part, a decimal point, and a decimal fraction part. In the following example, *16* represents the whole number part immediately before the decimal point. The numbers *4378* following the decimal point represent the fraction part. Since the last number *8* is in the ten thousandths column, the fraction represented is $^{4378}\!/_{10,000}$.

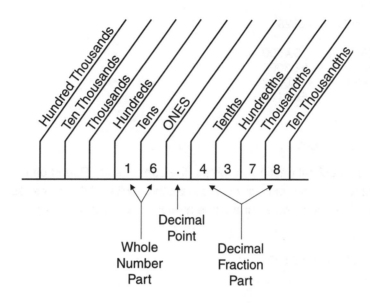

Rounding Off of Decimal Fractions:

Decimal fractions are rounded off for a specific degree of accuracy. If a decimal must be accurate to two places or to the nearest hundredth, first locate the number that indicates two places or hundredths. Increase the number by 1 if the number that follows it is 5 or more and then drop the remaining numbers. If the number that follows it is less than 5, simply drop all of the numbers that follow.

Example: Round off 16.4378 to tenths (one place after the decimal point).
Since the number after the 4 is 3, the numbers 378 are dropped.
16.4378 is rounded off to 16.4.

Example: Round off 16.4378 to hundredths (two places after the decimal point).
Since the number after the 3 is 7, one is added to the 3 to equal 4.
16,4378 is rounded off to 16.44.

Addition of Decimal Fractions:

To add decimal fractions, align all of the decimal points in a vertical column with the correct numbers placed before or after the decimal points in vertical lines. If there is no decimal point shown in a number, it is understood that the decimal point is to the right of the last digit. For example, the whole number 365 could be written as 365.0. Zeros can be inserted so all numbers have the same number of decimal places. Then add the numbers following the same rules used for addition of whole numbers.

Example: 3.45 + 52.3 + 0.0628

3.45	3.4500
52.3	52.3000
+ 0.0628	+ 0.0628
	55.8128

PRACTICAL PROBLEMS

1. Add the following decimal fractions to obtain the correct sum. Round off the answer to three decimal places or thousandths. (*Hint:* Add zeros as necessary so all numbers contain the same number of decimal places.)

    a. 5.893 + 87.32 + .5   _____

    b. 236.3421 + 92.17 + 56.647   _____

    c. 76 + 431.4996 + 3.22 + 0.5621   _____

    d. 8.0004 + .003 + 461.0247 + 105   _____

    e. 54.5 + .05455 + 5450 + 5.00456   _____

    f. 0.65 + 3,849.009 + 5.9863 + 372.90006   _____

2. A dental assistant (DA) orders the following supplies: 5 ounces (oz) of amalgam for $120.55, 1 box of composite for $54.79, 1 etch-prep kit for $33.64, 1 box of zinc oxide eugenol for $42.85, and 1 can of Lidocaine cartridges for $26.35. What is the total cost of the supplies?   _____

3. A public health nurse does a time breakdown for one day of work. If he spends 2.25 hours at the office, 0.75 hours traveling, 4 hours doing patient care, 0.25 hours on break, and 0.5 hours for lunch, what is the total number of hours?   _____

4. Five infants weighing 2.54 kilograms (kg), 4.045 kg, 3.3636 kg, 4.455 kg, and 3.2727 kg were born during one eight-hour shift. What was the total weight of the five infants?   _____

5. A medical assistant (MA) prepares a deposit slip for the bank. What is the total amount of money deposited?   _____

Coins	19	55
Currency	128	00
Checks:	2,139	95
	242	59
	83	60
	94	80
Total		
Less cash received		
TOTAL DEPOSIT		

6. If there are 15.5 grams (gm) of fat in a ham and cheese sandwich, 12.3 gm in 6 onion rings, 7.1 gm in a bag of potato chips, and 13.8 gm in a milkshake, how many grams of fat would this meal contain?   _____

7. A radiologist takes a series of X rays with the following quantities of radiation exposure: a chest film at 20.5 milliampere-seconds (mAs), a shoulder film at 15.5 mAs, and an upper arm film at 12.5 mAs. What is the total mAs of exposure?   _____

8. In a 24-hour period, an infant drinks 3.4 ounces (oz), 3.5 oz, 3.9 oz, 3.25 oz, and 3.75 oz of formula. How many ounces of formula did the infant drink?   _____

9. Calculate the bill for the following charges.   _____

SERVICE	CHARGE
Office visit	154.50
Blood test: CBC	89.78
Urinalysis	34.58
Medication	43.68
TOTAL	

10. An occupational therapy (OT) student pays $3,342.90 for tuition, $3,548.50 for room and board, $739.88 for books, and $17 for a parking sticker for one semester in college. What is her total cost?   _____

11. A registered dietitian (RD) calculates the sodium in the following breakfast: raisin bran cereal with 0.12 grams (gm), 1 cup 2% milk with 0.122 gm, 1 muffin with 0.37 gm, butter with 0.123 gm, and 1 glass of orange juice with .001 gm. How many gm of sodium are in the meal?   _____

12. A patient with pulmonary edema is given an initial dose of 0.04 grams (gm) of Furosemide at 9 AM. At 11 AM the patient receives another 0.04 gm, at 1 PM 0.06 gm, and at 7 PM 0.08 gm. What is the total dosage?   _____

13. A nutritionist creates a chart to show the amount of fiber in various foods.

DIETARY FIBER

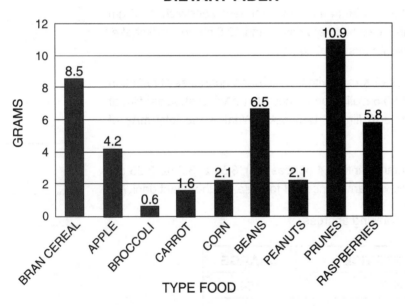

a. How many grams (gm) of fiber do the four vegetables contain?   _____

b. Does the bran cereal contain more or less fiber than the four vegetables?   _____

c. What is the total amount of fiber in all of the foods shown?   _____

14. A student saving for college has a balance of $3,942.56 in his savings account. During one month he deposits $50.75, $65.29, $47.68, and $54.14. At the end of the month $2.63 in interest is added to the account. What is the final balance? _____

15. A respiratory therapist (RT) uses a manometer to calculate oxygen usage at one-minute time intervals. She calculates that the following liters (l) are used: 1.883 l, 1.26351 l, 1.432 l, 1.98 l, and 1.87621 l. How many liters of oxygen were used? _____

16. A patient learning to use a prosthetic (artificial) leg walks 0.2 mile the first day. She then increases her distance by 0.2 mile each day.

    a. How many miles will she walk on day seven? _____

    b. How many total miles will she walk in one week (seven days)? _____

17. A patient is receiving Cytomel®, a thyroid preparation, for hypothyroidism. The first week she takes 0.025 milligram (mg) qd (every day). Each week the dosage is increased by 0.0125 mg until the desired effect is obtained. If it takes 5 weeks for her to obtain the right effect, what is her daily dosage during the fifth week? _____

18. A radiologist creates a chart showing the milliSieverts (mSv) of radiation exposure from various sources.

SOURCE OF RADIATION	mSv
Natural Sources:	
Radon	2.0
Cosmic Rays	0.28
Terrestrial	0.28
Body	0.39
Occupational Exposure	0.009
Nuclear Fuel Cycle	0.0005
Consumer Products	0.09
Miscellaneous Environmental	0.006
Medical Sources:	
Diagnostic X Rays	0.39
Nuclear Medicine	0.014

a. Do medical sources create more or less radiation exposure than natural sources? Why?   _____

b. If radon was eliminated, would medical sources contain more or less radiation exposure than natural sources?   _____

c. What is the exposure in mSv from occupational sources, consumer products, and miscellaneous environmental sources?   _____

d. What is the exposure in mSv from all sources shown? Round off the answer to three places or thousandths.   _____

Unit 12 SUBTRACTION OF DECIMAL FRACTIONS

BASIC PRINCIPLES OF SUBTRACTION OF DECIMAL FRACTIONS

To subtract decimal fractions, place the smaller number under the larger number with the decimal points aligned in a vertical column. Insert zeros as needed so both numbers have the same number of decimal places. Then subtract the numbers following the same rules used for subtraction of whole numbers. Be sure to put the decimal point in the same vertical position in the answer.

Example: 67.54 − 31.582

$$\begin{array}{r} 67.54 \\ -31.582 \\ \hline \end{array} \qquad \begin{array}{r} 67.540 \\ -31.582 \\ \hline 35.958 \end{array}$$

PRACTICAL PROBLEMS

1. Subtract the following decimal fractions. Round off the answer to two places or hundredths.

    a. 78.3 − 49.538   _____

    b. 0.5492 − 0.3629   _____

    c. 92 − 0.289   _____

    d. 123.824 − 79.55   _____

    e. 485.782 − 396   _____

    f. 3,586.3 − 2,978.564   _____

2. French fries cooked in beef tallow contain 18.5 grams (gm) of fat. If they are fried in vegetable oil, they contain 12.2 gm of fat. What is the difference?   _____

3. A patient has a bill for $15,109.61. Her insurance company pays $12,594.83. What is the balance?   _____

4. A one-year-old baby weighs 18.5 pounds (lb). At birth he weighed 6.75 lb. How much did he gain in one year?   _____

5. A medical laboratory technician (MLT) uses a refractometer to calculate the specific gravity of urine at 1.043. After the patient drinks a large quantity of fluids, the specific gravity is 1.028. What is the drop in specific gravity?   _____

6. A geriatric assistant checks his pay stub to note deductions taken out of his gross pay. What was his net pay?   _____

GROSS PAY	$289.60
Deductions:	
Federal Tax	$52.13
State Tax	$8.69
FICA	$22.15
City Tax	$4.34
NET PAY	

7. A patient's temperature is 103.6°F (Fahrenheit). After being given Tylenol, her temperature was 99.8°F. What was the drop in temperature?   _____

8. If a cup of whole milk has 8.2 grams (gm) of fat and a cup of skim milk has 0.4 gm, how much less fat does skim milk contain?   _____

9. A patient's hemoglobin was 17.5 grams (gm). After surgery, the hemoglobin dropped to 13.0 gm. What was the drop in hemoglobin?   _____

10. A physical therapist checks the temperature of water in a whirlpool tub and finds it is 35.6°C (Celsius). The water must be at 39.4°C. By how many degrees does the temperature need to be increased?   _____

11. A dentist studies the thermal conductivity (sensitivity to temperature) of tooth structures and materials used to restore the teeth.

THERMAL CONDUCTIVITY

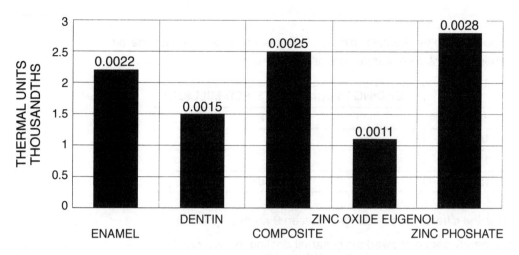

a. Would a layer of zinc oxide eugenol and composite have more or less thermal conductivity than the normal tooth tissues of enamel and dentin? What is the difference? _____

b. What would the difference be if zinc phosphate were used instead of the zinc oxide eugenol? _____

12. The maximum permissible dose (MPD) of radiation exposure for dental workers is 5 rem (radiation equivalent man). If a dental hygienist's dosimeter badge (device used to measure radiation) shows 2.8563 rem, how much more exposure can the hygienist have before reaching his MPD? _____

13. Human blood has a pH (measurement of acidity or alkalinity) of 7.4. A urine test shows a pH of 5.8 for the urine. What is the difference in pH between blood and urine? _____

14. A bacillus bacterium measure 8.6 micrometers (mcm) while a virus measures 0.07392 mcm. How much larger is the bacterium? _____

15. A genetic counselor at a prenatal (before birth) clinic has an annual budget of $168,429.82 allocated for amniocentesis tests (a test that checks for genetic defects in the fluid surrounding the unborn infant). At the end of June, $98,753.98 has been spent. How much money remains in the budget for tests?   _____

16. An occupational epidemiologist uses a toxic gas meter to evaluate the air after a chemical spill. She obtains the following results:

TIME	READING IN ppm (PARTS PER MILLION)
9:00 AM	765.798
10:00 AM	642.64
11:00 AM	533.7
12 Noon	416.836

a. What is the difference in readings between 9 AM and 12 Noon?   _____

b. Which hourly period showed the greatest decline in toxic gas?   _____

17. The number of Americans with high blood pressure increased to 92.31 million from 63.6 million ten years ago. In the same time period, the number of Americans with elevated cholesterol dropped from 49.4 million to 37.76 million after treatment with new medications. How many more people had an increase in blood pressure than a drop in cholesterol?   _____

18. The maximum safe environmental concentration of mercury (Hg) vapor in air
     is 0.05 milligrams (mg) of Hg per cubic meter of air for a 40-hour week. A
     dentist graphs the Hg vapor for various substances along with the measured
     Hg vapor in her office.

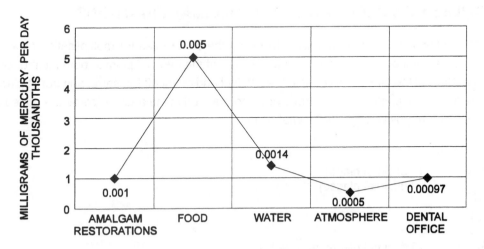

MERCURY VAPOR

a. How much greater is the total vapor from food, water, and the atmosphere
    than the vapor from amalgam restorations?   _____

b. How much greater is the vapor from two amalgam restorations than the
    vapor in the dental office?   _____

c. Is the five-day office level higher than the limit allowed? Why or why not?
    What is the difference between the two?   _____

Unit 13 MULTIPLICATION OF DECIMAL FRACTIONS

BASIC PRINCIPLES OF MULTIPLICATION OF DECIMAL FRACTIONS

To multiply decimal fractions, multiply the numbers following the same rules for multiplication of whole numbers. Then count the number of decimal places to the right of the decimal point in both the multiplier and the multiplicand. Start at the far right number in the product and count off the same number of places to the left before placing the decimal point. If extra places are needed in the answer, zeros are added on the left of the product before positioning the decimal point.

Example 1: 27.5 × 3.42

```
      27.5       (1 decimal place)
    × 3.42       (2 decimal places)
      550
     1100
      825
    94.050       (3 decimal places from right)
```

Example 2: 0.006 × 0.08

```
       .006    (3 decimal places)
     × .08     (2 decimal places)
    0.00048    (5 decimal places from right) (Note that zeros had to be added.)
```

PRACTICAL PROBLEMS

1. Multiply the following decimal fractions. Round off the answers to three decimal places or thousandths.

   a. 7.27 × 31.6 _____

   b. 28.561 × 5.39 _____

   c. 0.123 × 0.79 _____

   d. 73 × 2.14785 _____

   e. 0.614 × 0.00568 _____

   f. 82.005 × 5.98003 _____

2. A registered nurse (RN) buys five uniforms at $47.95 each. What was the total cost of the uniforms? _____

3. One breaded shrimp contains 0.9 grams (gm) of fat. How many gm of fat would one dozen shrimp contain?   _____

4. A biomedical equipment technician (BET) makes $728.25 per week. If she has to pay 0.0765 of the total amount to FICA (Social Security), how much is paid to FICA? (Round off to two places or hundredths.)   _____

5. One millimeter (mm) distance on ECG paper equals 0.04 seconds. How many seconds are represented by 75 mm?   _____

—1 SMALL BLOCK = 1 MILLIMETER
 1 MILLIMETER = 0.04 SECOND

75 MILLIMETERS

6. A patient takes 0.625 milligrams (mg) of Premarin® bid (twice a day) for five days. What is the total dose?   _____

7. A six-month-old infant weighs 8.41 kilograms (kg). If one kg equals 2.2 pounds (lb), how many lb does the infant weigh?   _____

8. A Red Cross disaster truck uses 0.053 gallons (gal) of gas per mile. During one year, the truck was driven 48,552 miles. If the average cost of gas was $1.449 per gal, how much was spent on gas? (Round off to two places or hundredths.)   _____

9. A person walking at a rapid pace burns 2.2 calories (cal) per pound (lb) qh (every hour). If a person weighs 142 lb and walks 1.25 hours, how many cal are burned?   _____

10. A respiratory therapist (RT) is trying to increase the humidity in the air. She knows that at 50°F saturated air contains approximately 4.2 grams (gm) of water per cubic foot of air. At 90°F, nearly 2.9 times as much water is retained. How much water is retained at 90°F in the room shown?   _____

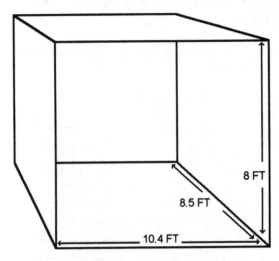

8 FT

8.5 FT

10.4 FT

CUBIC FEET = LENGTH x WIDTH x HEIGHT

11. A radiologist knows that when a radiographic tube is moved farther away the milliampere-seconds (mAs) must be increased while taking an X ray. He uses this formula:

$$\text{New mAs} = \frac{\text{Original mAs} \times \text{New SID}^2 \text{ (Source to Image Distance)}}{\text{Original SID}^2}$$

If the original mAs was 7.5, the original SID was 20 inches, and the new SID is 40 inches, what is the new mAs setting? (*Hint:* The SID must be squared as indicated by the ^{2}. For example, to square an SID of 10 inches, multiply $10 \times 10 = 100$ square inches.)   _____

12. The overall death rate for a population has been determined to be about 2.75 people per thousand people per year. In a population of 4,975,000 people, how many deaths would be expected in one year?   _____

13. A single Unopette® used for blood cell counts costs 58 cents. If a laboratory orders 16 dozen Unopettes®, what is the total cost?   _____

14. An intravenous (IV) solution of 5% D/W (Dextrose in water) is infusing at a rate of 1.75 milliliters (ml) per minute. How many ml would infuse in 7.5 hours?   _____

15. Statistics from the Centers for Disease Control and Prevention (CDC) show that between 0.223 and 0.2349 of adults over 20 years old are obese or overweight. The United States Census Bureau statistics state that 196,899,193 people are over 20 years of age. What is the range of people who are overweight? (Round off to the nearest whole number.) _____

16. A Healthy People study conducted by the United States government showed that 0.2785 of high school students smoked cigarettes. The same study showed that 0.2297 of adults smoked. If the adolescent population is 20,219,890, and the adult population is 209,128,094, how many smokers are there? (Round off to the nearest whole number.) _____

17. The allowable range for fluoride (Fl) in water is 0.7 to 1.2 parts per one million parts of water. If the United States uses 338 billion gallons of water per day, what is the range of Fl that could be used per day? _____

18. The American Cancer Society develops statistical multiplication factors to estimate various facts about cancer, shown on the following chart.

ESTIMATED CANCER STATISTICS

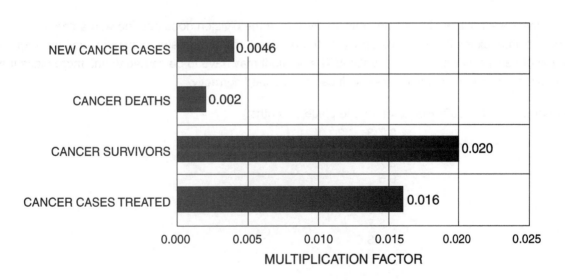

a. In a city with a population of approximately 248,000 people, how many new cancer cases are expected? _____

b. How many people will die of cancer in the same city? _____

c. In the same city, how many people will be under treatment and/or survivors of cancer? _____

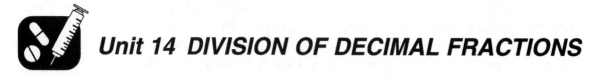

Unit 14 DIVISION OF DECIMAL FRACTIONS

BASIC PRINCIPLES OF DIVISION OF DECIMAL FRACTIONS

To divide decimal fractions, begin by placing the dividend (number to be divided) inside the division bracket and the divisor outside the bracket. Then convert the divisor to a whole number by moving the decimal point all the way to the right. Move the decimal point of the dividend the same number of places to the right. Put a decimal point in the quotient directly above the new placement of the decimal point in the dividend. Then follow the same rules for division of whole numbers.

Example: 13.68 ÷ 2.4

$$
\begin{array}{r}
5.7 \\
24.\overline{)136.8} \\
\underline{120} \\
168 \\
\underline{168}
\end{array}
$$

2.4)13.68

Note that the decimal points were moved one place to the right in the divisor and the dividend.

Remainders are not used in decimal fraction division. If the division does not end with a zero as shown in the previous example, zeros are added to the dividend and the division continues until the required number of decimal places is in the quotient. The quotient may have to be carried to one more place than the desired number of decimal places so it can be rounded correctly.

Example: 78.6 ÷ .09 (Round off to one place or tenths.)

.09)78.6

$$
\begin{array}{r}
873.33 \\
9\overline{)7860.00} \\
\underline{72} \\
66 \\
\underline{63} \\
30 \\
\underline{27} \\
30 \\
\underline{27} \\
30 \\
\underline{27} \\
3
\end{array}
$$

Answer: 873.3 rounded off to tenths.

Decimal points are moved two places in both the divisor and dividend. Three zeros are added to complete the division until it can be rounded to tenths.

PRACTICAL PROBLEMS

1. Divide the following problems. If necessary, round the answer to two places or hundredths.

    a. 125.49 ÷ 2.35 _____

    b. 411.768 ÷ 16.34 _____

    c. 78 ÷ 0.007 _____

    d. 30.58 ÷ 6 _____

    e. 5,892 ÷ 40.82 _____

    f. 6,420.3 ÷ 24.62 _____

2. A 12-ounce steak contains 14.04 grams (gm) of saturated fat. How many gm of fat are in each ounce? _____

3. A medical assistant (MA) buys 6 stethoscopes for $85.98. What is the cost of each stethoscope? _____

4. A physical therapist (PT) works 189.75 hours in 23 days. If she works the same number of hours per day, how many hours does she work per day? _____

5. A client at a weight loss clinic lost 23.75 pounds (lb) in 5 weeks. If he loses the same amount of weight each day, how much weight does he lose per day? (Round answer to three places or thousandths.) _____

6. How many grams (gm) of Ancef are in 1 milliliter (ml) of solution? _____

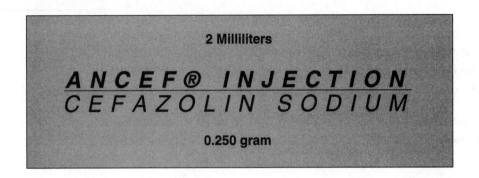

2 Milliliters

ANCEF® INJECTION
CEFAZOLIN SODIUM

0.250 gram

7. A dental laboratory technician (DLT) buys a case of Alginate containing one dozen cans for $138.36. What is the cost per can?   _____

8. A patient is taking 0.5 ounces (oz) of cough syrup per dose. If the bottle contains 16.5 oz, how many doses are in the bottle?   _____

9. A medical lab technologist (MT) buys 3.5 grams (gm) of sodium chloride (NaCl) to prepare a culture medium. If each culture requires 0.025 gm of NaCl, how many culture media can be made from the amount purchased?   _____

10. How many tablets of Lanoxin® should be given to a patient who requires a dosage of 0.25 milligrams (mg)?   _____

LANOXIN®

0.125 mg.

50 Tablets

11. A registered dietitian (RD) purchases 26.75 pounds (lb) of roast beef for $84.88. Each patient is served .25 lb.

    a. How many patients will the roast beef serve?   _____

    b. What is the cost per patient? Round off the answer to two places or hundredths.   _____

12. The United States Department of Health and Human Services (USDHHS) determined that 0.32 of adults studied had high blood pressure. If 6,328 people had high blood pressure, how many people were in the study? (*Hint:* Use 0.32 as the divisor.)   _____

13. A radiologic technician can purchase X-ray film at $74.76 for 24 exposures or $108.90 for 36 exposures. If both films are of equal quality, what is the best buy?   _____

14. An emergency medical technician (EMT) earns $9.97 per hour. One month she earns a gross pay of $1,951.63.

   a. How much did she make per week if it was a 4.5-week month? Round off answer to two places or hundredths. _____

   b. How many hours does she work per week? Round off answer to one place or tenths. _____

15. A patient on a low dose of aspirin (ASA) takes 17.5 grains (gr) per week. How many gr are in each tablet if the patient takes 2 tablets each day? _____

16. While taking X rays, grids are used at times to absorb scattered radiation. If a grid is used, 4 times more exposure in milliampere-seconds (mAs) must be used because part of the primary beam is absorbed by the grid. If 64.8 mAs are used with the grid, what was the mAs setting without the grid? _____

17. A hospital pharmacist is preparing potassium chloride (KCl) for injection. The vial states that there are 7.5 milliequivalents (mEq) of KCl per 5 millileters (ml) of solution. How many ml must be injected for a total dosage of 3 mEq of KCl? _____

18. A child weighing 46 pounds (lb) is put on Minocin®. The correct dose is .002 grams (gm) per kilogram (kg) of body weight. Round all answers to two places or hundredths.

---

60 Milliliters

MINOCIN® SUSPENSION
Minocycline Hydrochloride

0.050 gram in 5 milliliters

---

   a. How much does the child weigh in kg? (*Hint:* 1 kg equals 2.2 lb.) _____

   b. How many gm of Minocin® should the child receive? _____

   c. How many ml of Minocin® should be given to the child? _____

Unit 15 DECIMAL AND COMMON FRACTION EQUIVALENTS

BASIC PRINCIPLES OF DECIMAL AND COMMON FRACTION EQUIVALENTS

In order to work with both common fractions and decimal fractions, it is necessary to convert both numbers to either common fractions or decimal fractions.

To convert a common fraction to a decimal fraction, divide the numerator by the denominator. If the number does not come out even, it is usually rounded off to two or three places.

Example: Convert ¾ to a decimal fraction.

$$
\begin{array}{r}
.7 \\
4\overline{)3.00} \\
\underline{2\,8} \\
2
\end{array}
\qquad
\begin{array}{r}
.75 \\
4\overline{)3.00} \\
\underline{2\,8} \\
20 \\
\underline{20} \\
0
\end{array}
$$

To convert a decimal fraction to a common fraction, the number to the left of the decimal point is a whole number. The number to the right of the decimal point becomes the numerator of the common fraction. The denominator is determined by the place value of the last number after the decimal point. It will be 10 or a multiple of 10. The fraction is then reduced.

Example: Convert 2.625 to a common fraction.

2	.	6	2	5
Whole Number		Tenths	Hundredths	Thousandths
		10	100	1,000

$$2\,\frac{625}{1,000} \qquad \begin{array}{l}(625 \div 125 = 5) \\ (1,000 \div 125 = 8)\end{array} \quad = \quad 2\frac{5}{8}$$

PRACTICAL PROBLEMS

1. Convert the following common fractions to decimal fractions. Round off answers to three places or thousandths.

    a. $\frac{5}{16}$ _____

    b. $62\frac{2}{3}$ _____

    c. $43\frac{3}{5}$ _____

    d. $126\frac{15}{16}$ _____

2. Convert the following decimal fractions to common fractions.

    a. 23.8   _____

    b. 0.1875   _____

    c. 51.09375   _____

    d. 189.8125   _____

3. Express the temperature of 98.6°F (Fahrenheit) as a fraction.   _____

4. Write the formula for converting degrees Fahrenheit (°F) to degrees Celsius (°C) temperatures using a decimal fraction: °C = $\frac{5}{9}$ (°F −32)   _____

5. Write the formula for converting degrees Celsius (°C) to degrees Fahrenheit (°F) temperatures using a common fraction: °F = 1.8 °C + 32   _____

6. A patient is given $3\frac{1}{2}$ pints (pt) of blood. How many quarts (qt) of blood does this represent? Express the answer as a decimal fraction.   _____

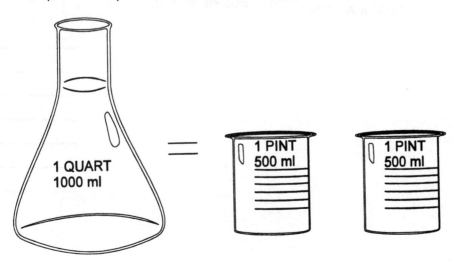

7. A disinfecting bleach solution contains 20 milliliters (ml) of bleach and 180 ml of distilled water for a total of 200 ml of solution.

    a. What common fraction represents the amount of bleach in the total amount of solution?   _____

    b. What decimal fraction represents the amount of distilled water in the total amount of solution?   _____

8. An infant is 21.875 inches (in) long. Write this as a common fraction.   _____

9. The pie chart shows the classifications of employees at City Hospital. Convert the decimal fractions to common fractions.

EMPLOYEES AT CITY HOSPITAL

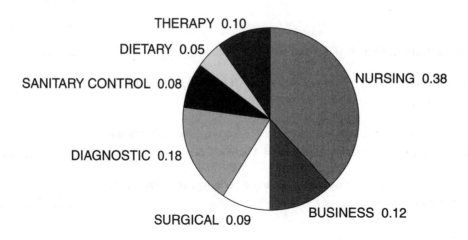

THERAPY 0.10
DIETARY 0.05
SANITARY CONTROL 0.08
NURSING 0.38
DIAGNOSTIC 0.18
SURGICAL 0.09
BUSINESS 0.12

    a. Business   _____
    b. Diagnostic   _____
    c. Dietary   _____
    d. Nursing   _____
    e. Sanitary Control   _____
    f. Surgical   _____
    g. Therapy   _____

10. City Hospital employs a total of 2,438 people. Use the pie chart in problem 9 to calculate the following. Round off all decimal fractions to a whole number.

   a. How many people are employed in nursing?   _____

   b. How many people are employed in diagnostic and therapy?   _____

   c. What common fraction would represent the difference between the total number of employees in nursing versus the total number of people employed in the business department?   _____

11. A bottle of cough syrup contains 36.5 ounces (oz). How many ¼-oz doses does the bottle contain?   _____

12. A patient with a heart condition calculates the miles he walks in one week. He walks 0.125 mile, ¼ mile, ⅓ mile, 0.375 mile, 0.1875 mile, ¾ mile, and ⅝ mile.

   a. How many miles did he walk expressed as a common fraction?   _____

   b. How many miles did he walk expressed as a decimal fraction? (Round to three places or thousandths.)   _____

13. A newborn infant weighs 8¾ pounds (lb). If 1 kilogram (kg) equals 2.2 lb, how many kg does the infant weigh? Express the answer as a decimal fraction rounded off to three places or thousandths.   _____

14. A diet consultant charts the weight loss for a client.

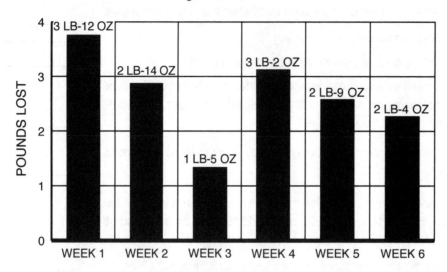

a. What is the patient's total weight loss in pounds and fractions of pounds? (*Hint:* 1 lb = 16 oz.)

_____

b. If the patient weighed 285.8 pounds at the start of the diet, how much does he weigh after 6 weeks?

_____

15. A patient is required to take 0.75 grams (gm) of a medication. The tablets are 0.5 gm. How many tablets should the patient take expressed as a common fraction?

_____

16. Is a specific gravity of urine of 1$\frac{3}{32}$ within the normal range of 1.010 to 1.025 for specific gravity? Why or why not?

_____

17. A microbiologist measures a bacterial specimen at 0.00163 micrometers (mcm) and a viral specimen at $\frac{13}{30,000}$ mcm.

a. Which specimen is larger, the bacterium or the virus?

_____

b. How much larger is the largest of the two specimens?

_____

18. The water line on a dental unit fits through a rubber tube that is lined with insulation to maintain the temperature of the water. If the water line has an outside diameter of 0.1875 inches (in), how thick is the layer of insulation? (*Hint:* Remember that the insulation is on both sides.)   _____

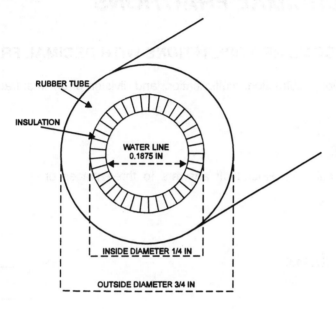

RUBBER TUBE

INSULATION

WATER LINE
0.1875 IN

INSIDE DIAMETER 1/4 IN

OUTSIDE DIAMETER 3/4 IN

Unit 16 COMBINED OPERATIONS WITH DECIMAL FRACTIONS

BASIC PRINCIPLES OF COMBINED OPERATIONS WITH DECIMAL FRACTIONS

Follow all of the rules for addition, subtraction, multiplication, and division of decimal fractions to solve the problems in this unit.

PRACTICAL PROBLEMS

1. Perform the operations indicated. Round off answers to three places or thousandths.

   a. $\dfrac{5.638 + .05327}{2.63}$ _____

   b. $4.56\,(32.901 + 63.2 - 27.9437)$ _____

   c. $(\dfrac{6.4}{2.2} \times 0.03) + 8.004$ _____

   d. $(48.1 - 30.006)\left(\dfrac{128.8 + 2.564}{3.09 - 0.58}\right)$ _____

2. The American Heart Association recommends that fat intake should be no more than 0.30 of daily calories (cal).

   a. If a person consumes 2,310 calories (cal) per day, how many cal of fat should the person consume? _____

   b. If there are 9 cal per gram (gm) of fat, how many gm of fat should the person consume per day? _____

3. A health care clinic has a real estate tax rate of $54.26 per thousand dollars of assessed value. If the clinic is assessed at $65,500.00, what is the real estate tax bill? _____

4. A normal oral body temperature is 98.6°F (degrees Fahrenheit). Use the formula to calculate the temperature in degrees Celsius (°C). _____

   $$°C = \tfrac{5}{9}\,(°F - 32)$$

5. A pediatric nurse (RN) orders 65 growth charts one month, 95 charts the second month, and 125 charts the third month. What was the total cost of the charts?   _____

PEDIATRIC GROWTH CHARTS PRICE LIST

Number of Charts	1–25	26–50	51–75	76–100	101–200
Price/Chart	$1.23	$1.12	$0.98	$0.80	$0.64

6. A licensed practical nurse (LPN) buys a uniform for $52.75, shoes for $63.49, and white support hose for $6.25. The sales tax rate is 0.0575 of the entire purchase. What was the total cost including sales tax?   _____

7. A public health department charges $5.00 for a flu shot. The vaccine costs $0.38 per shot, a syringe costs $0.14, and the labor cost for the nurse is $0.78 per shot. If 168 people get flu shots, what is the profit after all costs are subtracted?   _____

8. Statistics from the United States Department of Health and Human Services (USDHHS) show that the rate of suicide is 10.6 people per 100,000 population. In a city with 384,485 people, how many will commit suicide? Round off answer to one place or tenths. (*Hint:* First determine how many 100,000s there are in the total population.)   _____

9. A medical assistant (MA) orders supplies for the office. What is the total cost?   _____

QUANITY	UNITS	ITEM	COST PER ITEM	TOTAL COST
3	Cases	Latex Gloves	$27.65 per case	
2	Boxes	Tongue Depressors	$ 5.68 per box	
18	Each	Oral Thermometers	$12.60 per dozen	
6	Each	Rectal Thermometers	$12.60 per dozen	
24	Pints	Isopropyl Alcohol	$ 7.65 per dozen	
3	Boxes	Sterile Gauze	$ 4.95 per box	
			TOTAL	

10. An eight-year-old with convulsions is given Tridone®. For the first three days he receives 0.15 grams (gm) tid (three times a day). For the next three days he receives 0.225 gm tid. Tridone® is supplied in 0.150 gm tablets.

    a. What is the total daily dosage the first three days?   _____

    b. What is the increase in the daily dosage for the second three days?   _____

    d. How many tablets does he receive per day during the last three days? _____

11. A registered nurse (RN) working in the operating room earns $754.40 for a 40-hour week. A surgical technician earns $499.20 for a 40-hour week. What is the cost of labor for a 3½ hour surgery if one registered nurse and two surgical technicians are assisting?   _____

12. A child with asthma is given Aminophylline. The recommended dosage is 0.6 milligrams (mg) per kilogram (kg) of body weight. If the child weighs 54 pounds (lb), what dosage should she receive? Round off to one place or tenths. (*Hint:* 1 kg = 2.2 lb.)   _____

13. An athletic trainer (AT) is evaluating the differences between low- and high-intensity exercise for individuals with different weights.

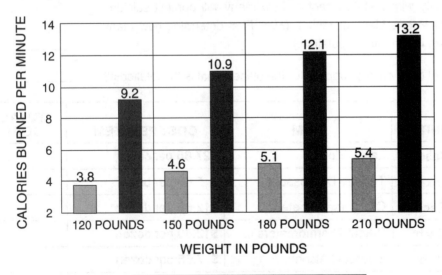

a. How many more calories (cal) will a 210-pound person burn in one hour doing high-intensity instead of low-intensity exercise?   _____

b. How many more cal will a 210-pound person burn than a 120-pound person if they both do high-intensity exercise for ½ hour?   _____

14. An emergency medical technician (EMT) earns $9.94 per hour. She works 40 hours plus 2.5 hours overtime which is paid at double time. Amounts deducted from her pay include 0.17 of the total pay for federal tax, 0.03 for state tax, 0.015 for city tax, and 0.0765 for FICA (Social Security). What is her take-home pay?   _____

15. An instructor is ordering supplies for a cardiopulmonary resuscitation (CPR) class. A package of 5 face masks costs $18.75 and a package of 10 airway bags costs $17.50. He must order full packages. Will the cost per student be higher if 9 students or 14 students take the class? What is the difference in the cost per student? Round off the answer to two places or hundredths.   _____

16. A hematologist is calculating the mean corpuscular hemoglobin (MCH) of a patient. If the patient has a red blood cell count (RBC) of 5,500,000 per cubic millimeter (mm) of blood and a hemoglobin (hgb) of 15.5 grams (gm), what is the MCH using the formula shown?   _____

$$MCH = \frac{\text{Grams of hgb}}{\text{RBC (millions/cubic mm)}} \times 10$$

17. A patient receives declining dosages of Prednisone over a 12-day period.

DAYS GIVEN	DOSAGE	TIMES PER DAY
Days 1–3	0.01 Gram (gm)	tid*
Days 4–5	0.005 gm	tid*
Days 6–7	0.005 gm	bid**
Days 8–9	0.0025 gm	bid**
Days 10–12	0.00125 gm	tid*

*tid = three times a day   **bid = twice a day

a. What is the total dosage for days 1–3?   _____

b. What is the decrease in total daily dosage between day 1 and day 12?   _____

c. What is the total dosage given to the patient in the 12-day period?   _____

18. A patient on a diet and exercise program loses 2.5 pounds (lb) the first week, gains 3.25 lb the second week, loses 1.25 lb the third week, loses 3.8 lb the fourth week, gains 1.75 lb the fifth week, and loses 4.3 lb the sixth week. If her original weight was 187¾ lb, what is her weight at the end of the six weeks?

    _____

19. An accountant is calculating the payroll for clinic employees. A receptionist earns $7.37 per hour, a licensed practical nurse (LPN) earns $12.46 per hour, two registered nurses (RN) each earn $18.32 per hour, and a technician earns $10.55 per hour. If they all work 38.5 hours, what is the total payroll? Round off all answers to two places or hundredths.

    _____

20. Statistics from the National Safety Council (NSC) show the number of deaths per 100,000 population from accidental causes by age group. A city has a total population of 431,620 people, of whom 0.06 are 0–4 years old, 0.12 are 5–14 years old, 0.18 are 15–24 years old, 0.21 are 25–44 years old, 0.24 are 45–64 years old, and 0.19 are over 65 years old.

ACCIDENTAL DEATH RATES

CAUSE OF DEATH	0–4 Years	5–14 Years	15–24 Years	25–44 Years	45–64 Years	Over 65 Years
Motor Vehicle	6.3	5.9	34.1	20.5	15.8	48.6
Drowning	5.7	1.4	2.5	1.8	1.3	0.09
Falls	1.3	0.8	0.2	1.4	3.2	68.0
Fire/Burns	3.9	0.9	0.8	1.1	1.6	8.8
Suffocation	11.3	0.6	1.0	4.0	1.7	15.4

Note: Death rates are shown per 100,000 population for each group.

a. In this city, how many more people over age 65 will die from falls compared to the total number of deaths from falls in all other age groups?

    _____

b. In the same city, what is the total number of people who will die in motor vehicle accidents?

    _____

c. In the same city, how many more people aged 15–25 die in motor vehicles than from all other types of accidental deaths shown?

    _____

d. What is the difference in the death rate per 100,000 population for all ages from suffocation compared to drowning?

    _____

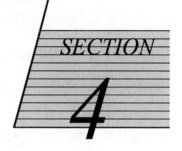

Percent, Interest, and Averages

Unit 17 **PERCENT AND PERCENTAGE**

BASIC PRINCIPLES OF PERCENT AND PERCENTAGE

Percent means the number of parts per one hundred. Twenty percent, written as 20%, means 20 parts out of 100 parts or $^{20}/_{100}$. Look at the following diagram and study what figures A, B, C, and D represent in the block of 100 squares.

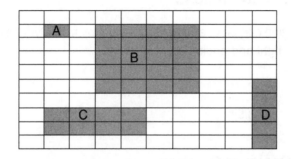

A = 1/100, 0.01, or 1% of total
B = 20/100, 0.20, or 20% of total
C = 10/100, 0.10, or 10% of total
D = 5/100, 0.05, or 5% of total

The previous figure clearly shows how a percent can be expressed as a common fraction or decimal fraction. To solve certain mathematical problems, it may be necessary to convert a percent to a common fraction or decimal fraction. The conversion can be done easily.

Converting a Percent to a Decimal Fraction:

Percent can readily be changed to a decimal fraction. To express a percent as a decimal fraction, divide by 100, or move the decimal point two places to the left and drop the percent sign.

Example 1: 28% = 28.% = 0.28

Example 2: 33.4% = 33.4% = 0.334

Example 3: 46⅕%   First change the ⅕ to a decimal by dividing the 1 by 5 to get 0.20.

46.2%   Write the percent with the decimal in place of the fraction.

46.2% = 46.2% = 0.462

Converting a Decimal Fraction to Percent:

In the same manner, a decimal fraction can be changed to a percent by multiplying by 100, or by moving the decimal point two places to the right and adding a percent sign.

Example 1: 0.56 = 0.56 = 56%

Example 2: 0.065 = 0.065 = 6.5%

Converting a Percent to a Common Fraction:

To change a percent to a common fraction, first change the percent to a decimal fraction. Then put the decimal fraction over the appropriate multiple of ten represented by the decimal fraction. Reduce the common fraction to lowest terms. Another method is to replace the percent symbol with 100 as the denominator of the fraction, and then reduce the fraction to lowest terms.

Example 1: 45 % = 45.% = 0.45 = $\dfrac{45 \ (^{45}\!/_5 = 9)}{100 \ (^{100}\!/_5 = 20)} = \dfrac{9}{20}$

Example 2: 40.8 % = 40.8% = 0.408 = $\dfrac{408 \ (^{408}\!/_8 = 51)}{1000 \ (^{1000}\!/_8 = 125)} = \dfrac{51}{125}$

Converting a Common Fraction to a Percent:

To convert a common fraction to a percent, first change the common fraction to a decimal fraction by dividing the numerator by the denominator. If a mixed number is involved, change the mixed number to an improper fraction first. Then convert the decimal fraction to a percent by multiplying by 100, or moving the decimal point two places to the right and adding a percent sign. Round off any numbers as indicated or as appropriate.

Example 1:

$$\frac{2}{5} = 5\overline{)\begin{array}{c} .4 \\ 2.0 \\ \underline{2\ 0} \\ 0 \end{array}}$$

$0.4 = 0.40 = 40\%$

Example 2:

$$1\tfrac{1}{2} = \tfrac{3}{2} = 2\overline{)\begin{array}{c} 1.5 \\ 3.0 \\ \underline{2} \\ 1\ 0 \\ \underline{1\ 0} \\ 0 \end{array}}$$

$1.5 = 1.50 = 150\%$

Note that the percent of 150% is greater than 100%. This is because the converted number is greater than one.

Percentage:

Percentage is the term used to describe the part of the whole number. It should not be confused with *percent* which has the symbol % attached to it. A formula frequently used is:

Percentage (part) = Percent (rate) × Base (whole)

The percent (rate) is written as a decimal. The base is the whole from which a part will be described as a percentage.

Calculating Percentage:

Calculating percentage means finding the part of a whole number. Use the formula shown and write the percent or rate as a decimal.

Example: What is 20% of 400? (*Hint:* The "of" means multiply.)

Percentage (part)	=	Percent (rate)	×	Base (whole)
Percentage	=	20%	×	400
Percentage	=	0.20	×	400
80	=	20%	of	400

Example 2:   What is 150% of 638?

Percentage	=	150%	×	638
Percentage	=	1.5	×	638
957	=	150%	×	638

Note that the answer of 957 is greater than 638. This is because 150% is more than 100%.

Calculating Percent or Rate:

When a problem asks for a rate, it is asking for a percent. To find rate, divide the percentage by the base. The quotient (answer) is then converted to a percent by multiplying by 100, or moving the decimal point two places to the right and adding the % symbol. The formula is as follows:

$$\text{Percent (rate)} = \frac{\text{Percentage (part)}}{\text{Base (whole)}} \times 100 \text{ (Then add \%.)}$$

Example 1:   What percent of 24 is 6?

$$\text{Percent} = \frac{\text{Percentage}}{\text{Base}} = \frac{6}{24} = 24\overline{)6.00} = .25 = 25\%$$

```
       .2 5
  2 4 )6 . 0 0
       4 8
       1 2 0
       1 2 0
```

Example 2: What percent of 82 is 20.5?

$$\text{Percent} \ = \ \frac{20.5}{82} \ = \ 82\overline{)20.50}$$

```
        .2 5
   82)2 0 . 5 0
      1 6 4
        4  1 0
        4  1 0
             0
```

$0.25 = 25\%$

Percent = 25%   Answer: 20.5 is 25% of 82.

Calculating the Whole or Base:

To find the base (whole) when the percent (rate) and percentage (part) are known, first change the percent to a decimal fraction. Then divide the percentage by the percent. Use the formula:

$$\text{Base (whole)} \ = \ \frac{\text{Percentage (part)}}{\text{Percent (rate) (Divide \% by 100 and drop \%.)}}$$

Example 1: 12 is 30% of what number? (*Hint:* First convert 30% to the decimal fraction of 0.30.)

$$\text{Base} \ = \ \frac{\text{Percentage}}{\text{Percent}} \ = \ \frac{12}{.30} \ = \ .30\overline{)12.00} \ = \ \frac{40.}{30\overline{)1200.}} \ = 40$$

```
30)1200.
   120
    00
```

Base = 40   Answer: 12 is 30% of 40.

Example 2: 56.4 is 40% of what number? (*Hint:* First convert the 40% to 0.40.)

$$\text{Base} \ = \ \frac{56.4}{0.40} \ = \ .40\overline{)56.40}$$

```
        1 . 4 1
   .40)5 6 . 4 0
      4 0
      1 6 4
      1 6 0
          4 0
          4 0
             0
```

Base = 141   Answer: 56.4 is 40% of 141.

PRACTICAL PROBLEMS

NOTE: For all answers, round off to two places or hundredths.

1. Perform the conversions indicated.

   a. Convert 39% to a decimal fraction.   _____

   b. Convert 0.653 to a percent.   _____

   c. Convert 65% to a common fraction.   _____

   d. Convert ⅜ to a percent.   _____

   e. Convert ⅖% to a decimal fraction.   _____

   f. Convert 180% to a common fraction.   _____

2. Solve the following problems involving percent and percentage.

   a. What is 20% of 3,560?   _____

   b. What is 6.5% of 645?   _____

   c. What is 125% of 865?   _____

   d. What percent of 640 is 40?   _____

   e. What percent of 880 is 220?   _____

   f. What percent of 535 is 88.5?   _____

   g. 144 is 15% of what number?   _____

   h. 175 is 35% of what number?   _____

   i. 331.768 is 22.6% of what number?   _____

3. A leukocyte (white blood cell or WBC) count determines that there are 8,742
   leukocytes per cubic millimeter (mm) of blood. If 36% of the leukocytes are
   lymphocytes, how many lymphocytes are in a cubic mm of blood?   _____

4. The human body contains 208 bones. The bones of the fingers and toes are
   called phalanges. Each thumb and each great toe contains 2 phalanges. All
   the other fingers and toes contain 3 phalanges each. What percent of the
   bones of the body are phalanges?   _____

5. Table salt (sodium chloride or NaCl) is 40% sodium (Na) by weight. If a box
   of salt weighs 26 ounces, how much Na is in the box of salt?   _____

6. During a one-year period, a hospital admits 1,526 patients with heart attacks.
   If this represents 28% of the patients admitted during the year, how many
   total patients were admitted to the hospital?   _____

7. The following pie chart shows emergency room admissions for a one-month period. A total of 1,364 patients were admitted.

EMERGENCY ROOM ADMISSIONS

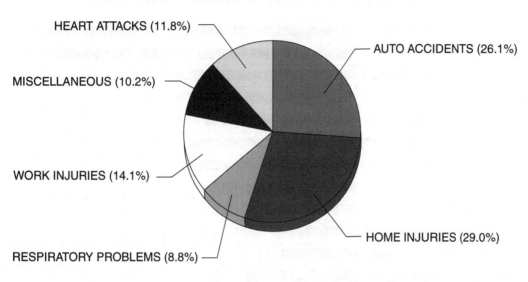

HEART ATTACKS (11.8%)

AUTO ACCIDENTS (26.1%)

MISCELLANEOUS (10.2%)

WORK INJURIES (14.1%)

HOME INJURIES (29.0%)

RESPIRATORY PROBLEMS (8.8%)

a. How many patients were admitted due to an injury at home or at work? _____

b. How many people were admitted with heart attacks or respiratory problems? _____

c. How many more people were admitted due to automobile accidents than were admitted with heart or respiratory problems? _____

8. Osteoporosis, a condition in which the bones become brittle and more likely to fracture or break, affects 25 million Americans. In one year, people with osteoporosis had 250,000 broken hips, 500,000 collapsing vertebrae, and 170,000 broken wrists. What percent of people with osteoporosis experienced fractures? _____

9. A doctor is building a new medical office building for a cost of $326,547. Building guidelines usually state that landscaping expenses should equal about 14% of the amount spent for the building.

a. How much should the doctor spend for landscaping? _____

b. What will the total cost of the building and landscaping be if the doctor spends the suggested amount? _____

10. A patient's bill for minor surgery is $3,858. Her insurance pays 82½%. How much must the patient pay?   _____

11. A survey on deficiencies of high school graduates indicates the problems shown on the graph.

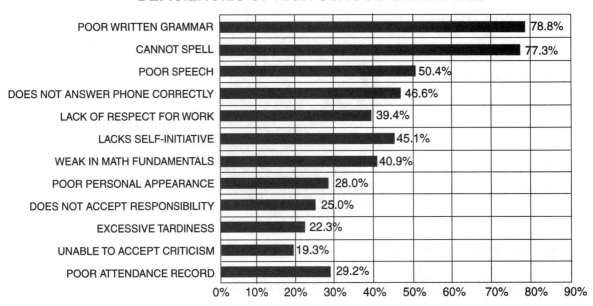

DEFICIENCIES OF HIGH SCHOOL GRADUATES

Category	%
POOR WRITTEN GRAMMAR	78.8%
CANNOT SPELL	77.3%
POOR SPEECH	50.4%
DOES NOT ANSWER PHONE CORRECTLY	46.6%
LACK OF RESPECT FOR WORK	39.4%
LACKS SELF-INITIATIVE	45.1%
WEAK IN MATH FUNDAMENTALS	40.9%
POOR PERSONAL APPEARANCE	28.0%
DOES NOT ACCEPT RESPONSIBILITY	25.0%
EXCESSIVE TARDINESS	22.3%
UNABLE TO ACCEPT CRITICISM	19.3%
POOR ATTENDANCE RECORD	29.2%

% OF COMPANIES REPORTING DEFICIENCY

a. What greater percentage of high school students exhibit poor written grammar as compared to poor speech?   _____

b. If a school graduates 594 students, how many could be expected to have poor written grammar?   _____

c. In the same school, how many students would be weak in fundamental math skills?   _____

12. The total cost for material and labor for performing a blood test is $76.28. If the laboratory adds 22³⁄10% for profit to this total cost, what is the charge for the blood test?   _____

13. A study shows an influenza (flu) vaccine is 71.4% effective in preventing a particular type of influenza. If 15,422 people receive the vaccine, how many would not be protected and would be likely to get influenza?   _____

14. Statistics from the Centers for Disease Control and Prevention (CDC) for a one-year period show 103,502 new cases of AIDS. If 9,279 of the cases are caused by heterosexual transmission, what percent of AIDS cases does this represent? _____

15. The pie graph shows the blood type by percentage for the general population of the United States.

BLOOD TYPES

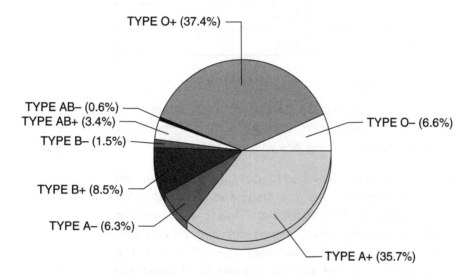

TYPE O+ (37.4%)

TYPE AB– (0.6%)
TYPE AB+ (3.4%)
TYPE B– (1.5%)

TYPE O– (6.6%)

TYPE B+ (8.5%)

TYPE A– (6.3%)

TYPE A+ (35.7%)

a. What total percent of the population has some type of Rh positive blood? (*Hint:* Rh positive is indicated by the "+" sign after the blood type.) _____

b. In a city with 549,623 people, how many people would have some type of Rh negative blood? _____

c. In the same city, how many people would have type O blood, either positive or negative? _____

16. In a survey of 51,321 high school seniors, 26% admitted to using marijuana at least once and 87% admitted to using alcohol.

a. How many students used marijuana? _____

b. How many more students used alcohol than marijuana? _____

17. Calculate a recreational therapist's net weekly pay by subtracting the percentages shown for various deductions from the gross weekly pay. (*Hint:* The percentages are all taken from the original gross pay.)

GROSS PAY		$742.63
DEDUCTION	PERCENTAGE	AMOUNT
Federal Tax	15%	
State Tax	$3\frac{3}{4}\%$	
City Tax	$1\frac{1}{2}\%$	
FICA (Social Security)	7.65%	
NET PAY		

18. Statistics from a one-year period show that 10,049 or 65% of the infants born with cerebral palsy had speech defects and mental retardation. How many infants were born with cerebral palsy in the one-year period?

_____

19. New federal guidelines have been established for determining hypertension (high blood pressure). Prehypertension is now diagnosed for any diastolic pressure (constant pressure when the ventricles are relaxed and filling with blood) from 80 to 89, and any systolic pressure (pressure when the ventricles are contracting and pushing blood into the arteries) from 120 to 139. The United States census shows a total of 196,899,193 people 21 years and older. Centers for Disease Control and Prevention (CDC) statistics show that 32.8% of this group have hypertension. How many people will be diagnosed with hypertension if an increase of 127% is expected over the current number of people diagnosed with hypertension?

_____

20. According to the *New England Journal of Medicine,* 54% of families agreed to donate organs from brain-dead patients between 1997 and 1999. Organ banks estimate that approximately 13,800 people die each year who are organ donor candidates. There are approximately 82,000 people on the nation's waiting list for transplants. What percent represents the deficiency between actual organ donors and people waiting for transplants?

_____

21. A pharmaceutical company is performing research studies on a new antibiotic. During the studies, $\frac{3}{8}\%$ of the people involved in the studies developed a rash and hives. If 802 people participate in the research studies, how many developed a rash and hives?

_____

22. The FICA deduction on gross pay includes payment for both Social Security and Medicare. The deduction for Social Security is 6.2% of any earnings up to a maximum of $87,900. The deduction for Medicare is 1.45% of all earnings. If the gross wages for one year are $88,946.56, what is the total amount deducted for FICA? _____

23. Diastole is the period of time when the ventricles of the heart are filling with blood. If the heart beats 75 times per minute, the duration of diastole is 500 milliseconds (msec). When the heart beats 180 times per minute, the duration of diastole is 125 msec. What is the percent of decrease in the duration of diastole when the heart beats faster? _____

24. The United States Department of Labor published the following projections for the American workforce.

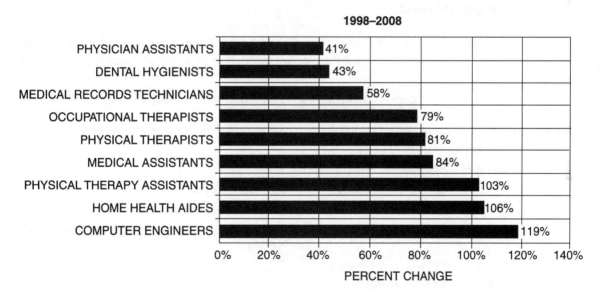

FASTEST GROWING OCCUPATIONS

1998–2008

a. How much greater is the percent change for home health aides than for dental hygienists? _____

b. Current employment figures for a state show 28,920 home health aides and 19,235 medical assistants. If the projections are correct, by the year 2008 how many more home health aides will there be than medical assistants? _____

c. The same state currently has 924 physical therapists and 1,256 physical therapy assistants. What will the total number of physical therapists and physical therapy assistants be in the year 2008 if projections are correct? _____

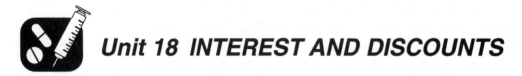 **_Unit 18 INTEREST AND DISCOUNTS_**

BASIC PRINCIPLES OF INTEREST

Interest and discounts are methods of using percent and percentage. Interest is usually charged when money is borrowed. The amount of money borrowed is called the _principal_. The charge for borrowing the money or principal is the _interest_. The _rate of interest_ is the percent used to calculate the interest due and is usually given for a one-year period of time. The _term_ is the length of time for the loan, usually based on years. The _amount_ is the total amount of money that must be repaid. It includes the principal plus the interest. When money is saved in a financial institution, such as a bank, interest is paid on the money saved. The same terms apply when interest is earned rather than paid.

Calculating Simple Interest:

Simple interest means that the rate of interest is calculated for the entire time period. The amount of interest is then added to the principal to find the amount owed. A formula for calculating _simple interest_ is:

$$\text{Interest} = \text{Principal} \times \text{Rate (expressed as a decimal fraction)} \times \text{Time}$$

Example: A college student borrows $3,000 for 1 year at an annual rate of 7%. What amount is due at the end of the year?

Interest = Principal × Rate × Time	
Interest = $3,000 × 7% × 1	(_Note:_ The 1 represents 1 year.)
Interest = $3,000 × .07 × 1	(Express the rate as a decimal fraction.)
Interest = $210.00	(This is the simple interest for the full year on the principal.)
Amount = Principal + Interest	
Amount = $3,000 + $210	
Amount = $3,210	(This is the total due at the end of one year.)

If the interest rate is based on one year, but the time period is more or less than one year, the time is written as a common fraction. Since there are 12 months in one year, a 6-month loan with an interest rate based on a one year period would use $^6\!/_{12}$ or $^1\!/_2$ or 0.5 for the time period. An 18-month loan would use $^{18}\!/_{12}$ or $^3\!/_2$ or 1.5 for the time period.

Calculating Compound Interest:

Compound interest is used more frequently than simple interest. *Compound interest* is interest based on the principal plus previously earned interest. If $500 is charged on a charge card with an annual interest rate of 18% compounded monthly, the amount due at the end of one month would be $507.50.

Example:

Interest =	Principal × Rate × Time	
Interest =	$500 × 18% × $^1\!/_{12}$	(*Note:* One month = $^1\!/_{12}$ or 0.083.)
Interest =	$500 × 0.18 × 0.083	(Express rate as a decimal fraction.)
Interest =	$7.50	(*Note:* This is interest for one month.)
Amount =	Principal + Interest	
Amount =	$500 + $7.50	
Amount =	$507.50	(This is the amount due at the end of one month.)

If no payment is made, the amount due at the end of the second month would show compound interest and would equal $515.11.

Example: $507.50 × .18 × $^1\!/_{12}$ = ?
$507.50 × 0.18 × 0.083 = $7.61
$507.50 + 7.61 = $515.11

Most car loans, home loans, and charge cards used compound interest instead of simple interest. In most cases, the interest is compounded daily. Computers or special calculators can quickly determine the amount due. Look at the following chart to see how $1,000 charged on a charge card can escalate when interest is compounded daily at a monthly rate of 1$^1\!/_2$% (yearly rate of 12 × 1$^1\!/_2$ = 18%). At the end of the month, the amount due is $1,015.10.

CALCULATING DAILY COMPOUNDING OF INTEREST

DAY	AMOUNT DUE	INTEREST CHARGE P × .015 × 1/30	AMOUNT + INTEREST
Day 1	$1,000.00	$0.50	$1,000.50
Day 2	$1,000.50	$0.50	$1,001.00
Day 3	$1,001.00	$0.50	$1,001.50
Day 4	$1,001.50	$0.50	$1,002.00
Day 5	$1,002.00	$0.50	$1,002.50
Day 6	$1,002.50	$0.50	$1,003.00
Day 7	$1,003.00	$0.50	$1,003.50
Day 8	$1,003.50	$0.50	$1,004.00
Day 9	$1,004.00	$0.50	$1,004.50
Day 10	$1,004.50	$0.50	$1,005.00
Day 11	$1,005.00	$0.50	$1,005.50
Day 12	$1,005.50	$0.50	$1,006.00
Day 13	$1,006.00	$0.50	$1,006.50
Day 14	$1,006.50	$0.50	$1,007.00
Day 21	$1,010.00	$0.51	$1,010.51
Day 30	$1,014.59	$0.51	**$1,015.10**

At the end of a period of time, the amount due will be greater if calculated with compound interest instead of simple interest. This is because the interest is not calculated on the principal alone, but on both the principal and the previous interest owed. However, financial institutions also give compound interest on savings, and many offer interest compounded daily for the benefit of the saver.

BASIC PRINCIPLES OF DISCOUNTS

A *discount* is an amount of money that is deducted from the cost. The *discount rate* is the percent by which the price is reduced. *List price* is the term used to describe the original cost of an item. *Net price* is the term used to describe the price of an item after the discount has been subtracted.

Two basic formulas are used to calculate discounts:

Discount = List Price × Discount Rate (expressed as a decimal fraction)

Net Price = List Price − Discount

Example 1: The list price for a stethoscope is $32 with a 12% discount for cash payments. What is the net price for a cash payment?

Discount =   List Price × Discount Rate

Discount = $32.00 × 12%

Discount = $32.00 × .12 = $3.84

Net Price =   List Price − Discount

Net Price = $32.00 − $3.84 = $28.16

Example 2: A physical therapist (PT) is ordering parallel bars. The list price of the bars is $786.48. A special sale offers a 15½% discount. If the bars are ordered by July 1st, an additional 12¼% discount can be taken on the net price. What is the final cost of the parallel bars?

Discount	= $786.48 × 15½%	Discount = List Price × Discount Rate
Discount	= $786.48 × 0.155	(Express rate as a decimal fraction.)
Discount	= $121.90	
Net Price	= $786.48 − $121.90	(Subtract the discount from the list price.)
Net Price	= $664.58	(*Note:* This is the discount on the list price.)
2nd Discount	= $664.58 × 12¼%	
2nd Discount	= $664.58 × 0.1225	(Express rate as a decimal fraction.)
2nd Discount	= $81.41	
Final Net Price	= $664.58 − $81.41	(Subtract the second discount.)
Final Net Price	= $583.17	(This is the final cost of the parallel bars.)

PRACTICAL PROBLEMS

NOTE: For all answers, round off to two places or hundredths.

1. Calculate the simple interest for the following:

   a. $5,400 borrowed at an annual rate of 7% for 2 years   _____

   b. $4,250 saved for 3 months at an annual rate of 3.5%   _____

2. Calculate the amount for the following:

   a. $820 borrowed for 3 months at an annual rate of 12% compounded monthly   _____

   b. $158 saved for 2 months at an annual rate of 4.5% compounded monthly   _____

3. Calculate the net price for the following discounts:

   a. List price of $58.80 discounted 25%   _____

   b. List price of $75.25 discounted 18.3%   _____

4. A bank loans a dentist (DDS) $7,500 for 1 year at a rate of 8¼% per year to purchase equipment. What is the yearly interest payment?   _____

5. A registered nurse (RN) borrows $3,590 for the purchase of a car. If he pays simple interest for 15 months at a rate of 7.5%, what amount will he owe at the end of the 15 months?

   _____

6. A sterile supply technician orders supplies totaling $1,234.56. She receives a 12% discount for payment within 30 days.

   a. If she pays within 30 days, how much of a discount will she receive?

   _____

   b. What is the final cost of the supplies?

   _____

7. A pharmacy technician student is buying books for his college courses. At the campus bookstore, the cost of the books is $878.52. At a Super Price bookstore, the cost of the books is $921.57 but they offer a 5¾% discount for a cash payment.

   a. If he pays in cash, which bookstore offers the better price?

   _____

   b. How much money does he save by paying in cash?

   _____

8. A medical laboratory buys a new computerized blood cell counter for $12,659.00. They receive a 15% discount for trading in an old model. They then receive an additional discount of 8.5% for payment within 30 days. What is the final cost of the blood cell counter?

   _____

9. An emergency rescue service makes the following purchase.

BILL OF SALE	AMOUNTS
Cost of New Ambulance	$ 189,954.28
Trade-in for Old Ambulance	$ 68,221.09
Down Payment	$ 37,500.00
Balance Due	
Interest on Balance	9.2 % Per Year
Term of Loan	2 Years

a. What is the balance due after the trade-in and down payment are deducted? _____

b. If the interest is compounded each year, what is the total amount of interest paid for two years? _____

c. If the total amount due at the end of two years is divided into monthly payments, what would each monthly payment be? _____

10. A geriatric assistant buys two new uniforms on sale. The first uniform lists for $47.59 with a 25% discount, and the second uniform lists for $58.95 with a 33% discount. He also has a coupon for 10% off the final total price of any purchase. What is his final cost for the two uniforms? _____

11. A student saving for college deposits an inheritance of $5,428.20 in a savings account. If the bank pays 3¾% interest per year compounded yearly, what will the balance be at the end of 2 years? _____

12. A surgical technician (ST) is purchasing sterile gloves. The gloves have a list price of $10.75 per box, but there is a sale with a 20% discount. If a case of 12 boxes is purchased, there is an additional 12% discount off the first net price. What is the net price for 3 cases of gloves? _____

13. A glucometer to check blood glucose or sugar levels costs $86.50. The company offers a $40 rebate. What percent of the cost is the rebate? _____

14. A respiratory therapist (RT) has a retirement account with a balance of $3,456.86. Each month 3% of her total paycheck is added to the account. In addition, her hospital contributes 2½% of the amount of her pay to the account. She is paid monthly on the first day of each month. If she earns $2,931.20 per month, and the bank pays 4.25% interest per year compounded monthly on the last day of each month, what will her balance be at the end of 2 months? _____

15. A physical therapist (PT) charges supplies on her charge card for a total of $4,328.86. The rate of interest is 18% per year compounded monthly. If she makes monthly payments of $150.00, how much would she owe at the end of three months?

_____

CALCULATION OF CHARGE CARD	AMOUNTS
Original Charge Amount	
+ Interest for First Month	
First Month Amount Due	
- Payment for First Month	
Amount for Second Month	
+ Interest for Second Month	
Second Month Amount Due	
- Payment for Second Month	
Amount for Third Month	
+ Interest for Third Month	
Third Month Amount Due	
- Payment for Third Month	
Final Balance After Three Months	

16. A medical office sends out bills for $746.35, $1,556.90, and $274.75 on January 1st with interest charged at a rate of 9% per year compounded monthly. If all three bills are paid in full on April 1st, with the correct amount of interest included, what is the total amount received?

_____

17. The net price for a refractometer to check specific gravity (SpGr) of urine is $342.50 after a 12% discount is allowed. What is the list price for the refractometer?

_____

18. A pharmacist is purchasing a new computer with a list price of $4,758.00. If she pays cash, she receives a 4% discount. She can also obtain a 1-year loan with a rate of 8.5% per year, a 2-year loan with a rate of 7.25% per year, or a 3-year loan with a rate of 4.75% per year.

   a. What is the least expensive loan in relation to the total amount of interest paid?   _____

   b. What is the difference in cost between paying cash or taking the least expensive loan?   _____

19. A dental laboratory orders supplies for a total of $6,439.65. A 6¼% discount is given if payment is made within 15 days, and a 2.5% discount is given if payment is made within 30 days. How much money can be saved by paying in 15 days instead of 30 days?   _____

20. A medical student borrows $18,300 at a rate of 4.5% per year compounded yearly for four years of medical school. After graduating, she must begin repaying the loan by paying 10% of her monthly income. She earns $73,538 per year.

   a. What is the amount due at the end of 4 years?   _____

   b. What is her monthly payment on the loan?   _____

   c. If interest is added at the end of each year to the amount still due, how long will it take her to repay the loan?   _____

Unit 19 AVERAGES AND ESTIMATES

BASIC PRINCIPLES OF AVERAGES

An average is a number that is representative of a group or *set* of numbers. There are different types of averages. One of the most common is the *arithmetic mean.* It is calculated by adding all of the numbers in the set and then dividing the sum by the number of units or values added. For example, the average or arithmetic mean of six numbers is the sum of the numbers divided by 6.

There are other types of averages. The *median* average is a positional number where average represents the middle number in a set of numbers. For example, in the set 20, 22, 24, 26, and 28, the median average is *24,* or the number in the middle. The *mode* average is the number or numbers that occur most frequently in a set. For example, in the set 22, 28, 26, 22, 24, the mode average is *22,* or the number that occurs most frequently in the set. Some sets will not have a mode. Since the mean average is the one used most frequently, any questions relating to "average" will ask for the "mean average."

Example: Find the average percent on a test if grades were 78%, 87%, 98%, 64%, and 91%.
(*Note:* 5 grades equal 5 units.)

78% + 87% + 98% + 64% + 91% = 418%
418% ÷ 5 (number of units) = 83.6% is the average percent

It is important to note that all of the units averaged must be the same unit of measure. In the example, all units are percents. To average ½, 0.65, 0.8, and ¾, the units must first all be converted to decimal or common fractions.

Example: ½ + 0.65 + 0.8 + ¾ =
0.5 + 0.65 + 0.8 + 0.75 = 2.7   (Convert all units to decimal fractions.)
2.7 ÷ 4 = 0.675   (Divide the sum by the number of units or 4.)

Averages can also be used to determine an unknown quantity. A student has test scores of 94%, 88%, and 84%. The student wants to know what score he must get on the final exam to have an overall average of 90%. Multiply the average desired by the total units, and then subtract the sum of the known units to get the unknown unit.

Example: 90% (average desired) × 4 (total number of tests) = 360%
94% + 88% + 84% (three known quantities) = 266%
360% (desired quantity) − 266% (known quantity) = 94%

The student must get a 94% on the fourth test to have an overall average of 90%.

BASIC PRINCIPLES OF ESTIMATES

An estimate is similar to an average, but it represents an approximate quantity. Estimates do not always represent exact numbers. For example, a cytologist is an individual who studies cells on slides. In a four-hour period of time, a cytologist examines 12 slides the first hour, 16 slides the second hour, 11 slides the third hour, and 14 slides the fourth hour. By adding the four numbers together and dividing by 4, it is possible to determine the average number of slides the cytologist examines per hour.

Example: 12 + 16 + 11 + 14 = 53 ÷ 4 = 13.25

After obtaining this average, an estimate could be given that this cytologist will examine 13.25 or 13 slides during the fifth hour. However, this is only an estimate since the cytologist may examine more or less slides depending on how complicated each slide is. In this manner, the estimate provides the best information available.

Estimates can be useful in planning. For example, an estimate can be made for the approximate number of slides the cytologist could examine in an 8-hour day. The estimate shows that 13.25 slides can be examined per hour. In an 8-hour period, the cytologist could examine 106 (8 × 13.25) slides. This estimate could be used to plan the daily work load of the cytologist. This does not mean that the cytologist will examine 106 slides in one day. She may examine more or less slides. However, the estimate is a good approximation of what could occur.

PRACTICAL PROBLEMS

Note: For all problems, round off to two places or hundredths.

1. Find the mean averages for the following groups of numbers.

    a. 38, 56, 45, 41, and 59 _____

    b. $52.55, $48.32, $43.97, and $41.61 _____

    c. 76%, 85%, 94%, 83%, 78% _____

    d. 56.6 mm, 48.2 mm, 61.8 mm _____

    e. 32.5 in, 24$\frac{3}{4}$ in, 36$\frac{3}{8}$ in, 22.25 in, 40$\frac{5}{8}$ in _____

    f. 6 pounds (lb) 4 ounces (oz), 8 lb 5 oz, 9 lb 14 oz, 7$\frac{1}{4}$ lb (*Hint:* 16 oz = 1 lb.) _____

2. A student receives test scores of 96%, 72%, 85%, and 91%. What is the average test score? _____

3. A microhematocrit (hct) measures the percent of erythrocytes (red blood cells or RBCs) in blood. To perform a microhematocrit, two tubes are filled with blood and centrifuged to allow the red blood cells (RBCs) to settle at the bottom of the tube. Then the percent of RBCs is calculated. The two readings are averaged to obtain the hct reading.

    a. If the tubes measure 32% and 28%, what is the hct? _____

    b. If the tubes measure 39% and 42%, what is the hct? _____

4. A dental hygiene student uses the Internet for research. He accesses the Internet through a local online provider. During one week, his online time is 32 minutes, 54 minutes, 27 minutes, 43 minutes, 21 minutes, 19 minutes, and 49 minutes.

    a. What is the average daily online time? _____

    b. If the online service charges $0.04 per minute, what is the student's average daily cost? _____

    c. In a 30-day month, what is the student's estimated monthly cost for the online Internet provider service? _____

5. The average daily sodium intake of a group of nurses is calculated and recorded. The amounts are 2120 milligrams (mg), 2932 mg, 1856 mg, 3688 mg, 853 mg, 3421 mg, and 1479 mg.

    a. What is the average daily sodium intake?   _____

    b. If the recommended normal sodium intake is 1100 mg to 3300 mg per day, does the average fall within normal limits?   _____

6. The length of different viruses is measured in micrometers (mcm) ($\frac{1}{1000}$ of a millimeter). What is the average length?   _____

LENGTHS OF VIRUSES

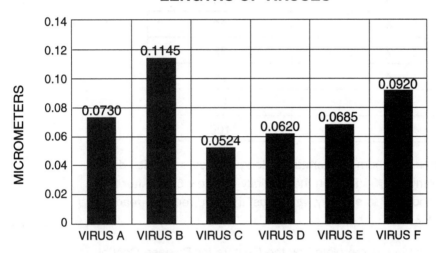

7. A diabetic checks his blood glucose level qid (four times a day) and obtains the following readings: 92 milligrams (mg), 123 mg, 125 mg, and 138 mg.

    a. What is the average reading for blood glucose?   _____

    b. If the normal range for blood glucose is 80–120 mg, does the average fall within normal limits?   _____

8. A medical accountant checks the electric bills for a medical clinic for a 6-month period. The bills are $178.34, $165.97, $192.91, $183.26, $173.44, and $168.75. To prepare an annual budget for the clinic, what amount should she use as an estimate for the cost of electricity per year?   _____

9. To perform an erythrocyte (red blood cell or RBC) count, 5 areas on a hemacytometer chamber are counted. If the counts are 101, 99, 105, 98, and 102, what is the average number of erythrocytes per area?   _____

10. A class of health occupations students received the test scores shown on an anatomy and physiology test. What is the average score?   _____

NUMBER OF STUDENTS	TEST SCORE
1	55
3	60
2	65
0	70
5	75
4	80
7	85
4	90
2	95
1	100

11. Federal law requires that room temperature in long-term care facilities does not exceed a maximum of 84°F when the humidity is below 60%. After two readings of 83°F and 86°F in one day, what must the third required reading be to average 84°F?   _____

12. The death rate for infants is calculated by the Centers for Disease Control and Prevention (CDC). In one year, the rate for white infants was 5.7, the rate for African American infants was 13.5, the rate for Asian or Pacific Islander infants was 4.9, the rate for Hispanics infants was 5.6, and the rate for infants of other races was 13.6. All of the rates were per 1,000 live births. What was the average rate for all races per 1,000 live births?   _____

13. In a three-year period, the CDC reported the number of pregnant women who tested positive for the HIV or AIDS virus. The first year showed 1.7, the second year showed 1.8, and the third year showed 1.4 women per 1,000 women tested. If 450,000 women are tested in the fourth year, what estimated number of women will have a positive test?   _____

14. A pediatric nurse (RN) records the weights of infants born during one day. What is the average weight of the infants born? (*Hint:* There are 16 ounces (oz) in 1 pound (lb). Remember, all units must be the same before an average can be calculated.)   _____

WEIGHT OF INFANTS

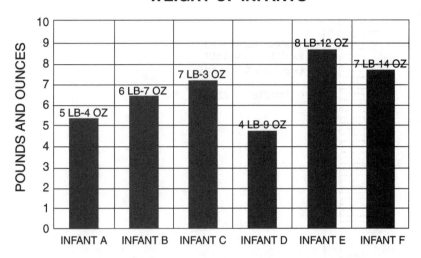

15. A radiology student is taking a math course and has had two tests with grades of 87% and 92%, each worth 25% of his final grade. He still has to take the final test which is 50% of his grade. What grade must he receive on his final to receive a 93% or A as a final grade?   _____

16. The National Highway Traffic Safety Administration publishes figures that show that 64% of pedestrian deaths occur at night, 53% occur on a weekend, and 35% of the pedestrians are intoxicated. If there are 15,546 pedestrian deaths in one year, what estimated number were intoxicated and killed on a weekend night?   _____

17. A health department receives state and federal grants for various programs. In one year, they receive grants for $94,076 for HIV/AIDS testing, $54,080 for cancer screening, $67,480 for health assessments, $67,276 for child health services, $111,120 for home health care, $45,836 for immunizations, and $19,163 for lead poisoning prevention. What is the average amount for grants?   _____

18. An erythrocyte sedimentation rate (ESR) measures the rate at which red blood cells settle in a tube. Readings taken at 15-minute intervals are shown on the diagram. What is the average rate of fall per 15-minute period?   _____

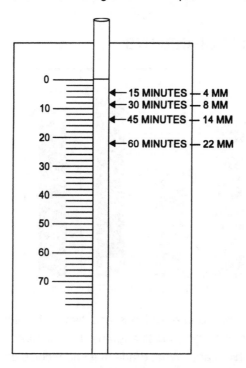

19. The National Head Injury Foundation estimates that every 15 seconds someone in the United States will suffer a traumatic brain injury, that approximately 750,000 people per year require hospitalization for such an injury, and that approximately 123,000 people die of such injuries.

   a. How many estimated head injuries occur every day?   _____

   b. Approximately how many people per day will require hospitalization?   _____

   c. Approximately how many people will die each day?   _____

20. The American Heart Association estimates that 1.5 million Americans will have heart attacks in one year, and that about 35% will die. If better health care and healthier living habits can cause a decrease in the number of heart attacks by 4% per year, how many deaths will there be from heart attacks per year at the end of the third year?   _____

21. A physical therapy student is budgeting for college. She bought 5 books for $432.56 the first semester, 3 books for $296.32 the second semester, 4 books for $387.39 the third semester, and 4 books for $355.21 the fourth semester. How much should she budget for books if she needs 5 books the fifth semester?   _____

Ratio and Proportion

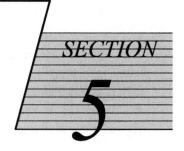

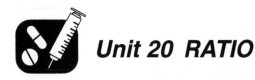

Unit 20 RATIO

BASIC PRINCIPLES OF RATIO PROBLEMS

A ratio is the comparison of one quantity with another similar quantity. The quantities that are compared are the *terms* or *components* of the ratio. The components are usually written with a colon (:) or the word "to" between them. They can also be written as a fraction. For example, if a class contains 12 boys and 14 girls, the ratio of boys to girls in the class can be written as 12:14, 12 to 14, or $^{12}/_{14}$. The terms or components are usually expressed in their lowest terms. In the previous example, both 12 and 14 can be divided by 2 to reduce the numbers to their lowest terms. The ratio of boys to girls would then be expressed as 6:7, 6 to 7, or $^6/_7$. It is important to remember that all terms must be similar. If container A holds 3 quarts and container B holds 1 gallon, the ratio would not be 3:1. The gallon would have to first be changed to 4 quarts. The ratio would then be 3:4.

Example: A supply cabinet contains 24 rectal thermometers and 60 oral thermometers. What is the ratio of oral thermometers to rectal thermometers?

The number of oral to rectal thermometers must be in the correct order:

60:24   or   60 to 24   or $^{60}/_{24}$

Both 60 and 24 can be divided by 12.

$60 \div 12 = 5$ $24 \div 12 = 2$

The ratio is then expressed in lowest terms.

5:2   or   5 to 2   or $^5/_{12}$

PRACTICAL PROBLEMS

1. Express the ratios in lowest terms.

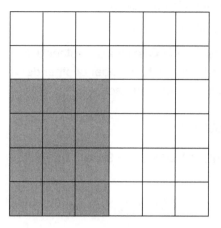

   a. Ratio of shaded squares to total squares

   _____

   b. Ratio of shaded squares to unshaded squares

   _____

   c. Ratio of unshaded squares to shaded squares

   _____

   d. Ratio of unshaded squares to total squares

   _____

2. To mix an ultrasonic cleaning solution, 10 milliliters (ml) of concentrated cleaner is added to 500 ml of distilled water. What is the ratio of cleaner to water?

   _____

3. A differential count of white blood cells counts 5 monocytes in a total of 100 leukocytes (white blood cells or WBCs). What is the ratio of monocytes to total leukocytes?

   _____

4. The label on a gallon of ice cream shows the total fat contents as 12 grams (gm) of which 8 gm is saturated fat. What is the ratio of saturated fat to total fat?

   _____

5. The peripheral nervous system (PNS) connects to the brain and spinal cord by 12 pairs of cranial nerves and 31 pairs of spinal nerves. What is the ratio of cranial nerves to the total number of nerves? (*Hint:* Note that the numbers are given as "pairs.")

   _____

6. To dilute blood for a leucotyte (white blood cell or WBC) count, 0.5 units of blood is added to 10 units of diluting solution. What is the ratio of blood to diluting solution?

   _____

7. At a city hospital, doctors performed 48 Caesarean sections (C-sections) out of a total 168 infants delivered.

    a. What is the ratio of C-sections to total infants delivered?   _____

    b. What is the ratio of C-sections to other deliveries?   _____

    c. For every 1 C-section, what is the ratio of C-sections to other deliveries? (*Hint:* Divide the number of C-sections into the number of other deliveries. Then express the ratio as 1 to the answer obtained.)   _____

Use the following figures to complete problems 8–10.

CANCER DEATHS BY SITE AND SEX

Male	Female
Lung & bronchus 89,200 (31%)	Lung & bronchus 65,700 (25%)
Prostate 30,200 (11%)	Breast 39,600 (15%)
Colon & rectum 27,800 (10%)	Colon & rectum 28,800 (11%)
Pancreas 14,500 (5%)	Pancreas 15,200 (5%)
Non-Hodgkin's Lymphoma 12,700 (5%)	Ovary 13,900 (5%)
Leukemia 12,100 (4%)	Non-Hodgkin's Lymphoma 12,700 (4%)
Esophagus 9,600 (3%)	Leukemia 9,600 (4%)
Liver 8,900 (3%)	Uterne corpus 6,600 (2%)
Urinary bladder 8,600 (3%)	Brain 5,900 (2%)
Kidney 7,200 (3%)	Multiple myeloma 5,300 (2%)
All Sites 288,200 (100%)	All Sites 267,300 (100%)

8. What is the ratio of deaths from lung cancer in males to deaths from lung cancer in females?   _____

9. What is the ratio of deaths from breast cancer in females to deaths from all sites in females?   _____

10. What is the ratio of deaths in males from prostate, colon, and rectum cancer to deaths from ovary and uterus cancer in females?   _____

11. A dental worker has a maximum permissible dose (MPD) of radioactive exposure of 5 rem per year. For the general public, the MPD is 0.5 rem per year. What is the ratio of rem allowed for the general public compared to that for a dental worker?   _____

12. A small laboratory beaker holds 50 milliliters (ml) of solution. A large graduate holds 2 liters (l). What is the ratio of the holding capacity of the large graduate compared to that of the small beaker. (*Hint:* 1 l = 1000 ml.)   _____

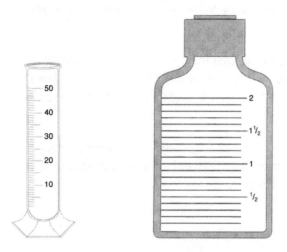

13. A study showed the chicken pox vaccine can save $5 for every $1 in cost. If 26,400 children are immunized at a cost of $35 per child, how much money would be saved?   _____

14. American Cancer Society statistics show that between 1983 and 1999, smoking among college graduates decreased from 21% to 11%. In adults without a high school education, the percentage decreased from 41% to 32%.

   a. What is the ratio for the percentage of college graduates who do not smoke now to the percent of adults without a high school education who do not smoke now?   _____

   b. What is the ratio for the percent of decrease in college graduates to the percent of decrease in adults without a high school education? (*Hint:* To find the percent of decrease, calculate the difference between the high rate and the low rate. Then divide the difference by the high rate.)   _____

15. National Safety Council statistics show that a death is caused by a motor vehicle crash every 12 minutes. Every 14 seconds a disabling injury is caused by a motor vehicle crash. What is the ratio of deaths to disabling injuries? (*Hint:* Express deaths as 1:? or 1 to ?.)

       _____

16. A state's health department compiles statistics showing a total of 2,698 people tested positive for the HIV virus causing acquired immune deficiency syndrome (AIDS). A total of 28,720 people were tested. Express this as a ratio of positive cases to negative cases with the positive cases expressed as 1. (*Hint:* Ratio must be shown as 1:? or 1 to ?.)

       _____

17. A solution of boric acid is mixed at a 1:20 ratio. If there are 1,000 milliliters (ml) of distilled water in the solution, how many ml of boric acid are present? (*Hint:* A 1:20 ratio means there is 1 ml of boric acid for every 20 ml of distilled water.)

       _____

18. A bleach disinfecting solution is mixed at a 2:5 ratio. If the solution has 0.5 liters (l) of distilled water, how many milliliters (ml) of bleach does it contain. (*Hint:* Convert the liters (l) to milliliters (ml).)

       _____

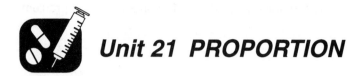 **Unit 21 PROPORTION**

BASIC PRINCIPLES OF PROPORTION PROBLEMS

A proportion is an equation that states that two ratios are equal. It is written with an equal sign between two ratios. An example might be 1:2 = 3:6. The first and last numbers of the proportion, in this case the 1 and 6, are called the *extremes* and the two middle numbers, the 2 and 3, are called the *means*. In order for a proportion to be a true proportion, the product of the means must equal the product of the extremes.

Example: Is 1:2 = 3:6?

Multiply the means: $2 \times 3 = 6$

Multiply the extremes: $1 \times 6 = 6$

Since 6 = 6, this is a true proportion.

If one factor in a true proportion is unknown, it is easy to find out what the factor is since the product of the means must equal the product of the extremes.

Example: How many milligrams (mg) of medication would you give an 80-pound person if you should give 20 mg for every 10 pounds?

$$\frac{20 \text{ mg}}{10 \text{ lb}} = \frac{X \text{ mg}}{80 \text{ lb}}$$ (*Note:* "*X*" represents the unknown.)

Write as a proportion: 20:10 = *X*:80

Multiply the means: $10 \times X = 10X$

Multiply the extremes: $20 \times 80 = 1600$

Write as means equals extremes: $10X = 1600$

Divide both sides by 10 to solve for *X*:

$10X/10 = X$ $1600/10 = 160$

Write the answer: $X = 160$ mg (*Note: X* equals mg.)

Some people find it easier to use cross-multiplication to solve proportions. To solve the same problem with cross multiplication, follow these steps.

$$\frac{20}{10\ lb} = \frac{X\ mg}{80}$$

Cross-multiply as indicated by the arrows:

$10 \times X = 10X$ $20 \times 80 = 1600$

Write as two products equaling each other: $10X = 1600$

Divide both sides by 10 to obtain the value for X: $\frac{10X}{10} = \frac{1600}{10}$

$X = 160$ mg

Answer: An 80-pound person needs 160 mg of the medication.

Proportions can also be used while preparing solutions. For example, a 10% bleach solution means that there are 10 parts of bleach for every 100 parts of solution. The 10% is written as 0.10 or $\frac{10}{100}$ or a ratio of 10:100 reduced to 1:10. Any percent can be converted to a ratio.

Example: How many grams (gm) of boric acid crystals are needed to prepare 500 milliliters (ml) of a 5% boric acid solution?

First calculate that a 5% boric acid solution equals 0.05 or $\frac{5}{100}$ or 5:100 or 1:20. This means there is 1 gm of boric acid crystals in every 20 ml of solution.

Next, set up a proportion:

$$\frac{1\ gm}{20\ ml} = \frac{X\ gm}{500\ ml}$$ (unknown quantity) (quantity desired)

Multiply the means: $20 \times X = 20X$

Multiply the extremes: $1 \times 500 = 500$

Write as means equals extremes: $20X = 500$

Divide both sides by 20 to find X:

$20X/20 = X$ $500/20 = 25$

Write the answer: $X = 25$ gm   (Use 25 gm of boric acid.)

PRACTICAL PROBLEMS

1. Solve for the *X* in the following proportions:

    a. 300 mg:1 tablet = *X* mg:3 tablets   _____

    b. 250 mg:5 ml = 125 mg:*X* ml   _____

    c. 15 ml:250 ml = *X* ml:1000 ml   _____

    d. gr ¼:1 tablet = gr ⅛:*X* tablets   _____

2. To mix plaster for a dental model, 45 milliliters (ml) of water are used for 100 grams (gm) of plaster. How many ml of water should be used for 200 gm of plaster?   _____

3. A CPR instructor is preparing a 10% bleach solution (bleach in distilled water) to clean the CPR manikins. How many milliliters (ml) of distilled water should she use to prepare 50 ml of bleach solution?   _____

4. A patient is to receive 50 milligrams (mg) of Demerol. Tablets available are 25 mg. How many tablets should the patient take?   _____

5. One millivolt (mV) of electricity causes the stylus on an electrocardiograph (ECG) machine to move 10 millimeters (mm) vertically. How many mm would the stylus move with 3.5 mV of electricity?   _____

6. A laboratory technician can clean 45 pipettes every hour with an automatic washer. How many can he clean in 15 minutes? (*Hint:* Both time periods must be in the same unit of measurement.)   _____

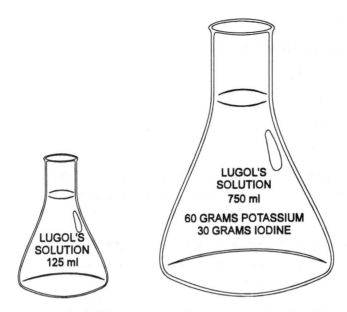

Use the diagram for problems 7 and 8.

7. How many grams (gm) of potassium (K) are required for 125 milliliters (ml) of Lugol's solution?   _____

8. How many gm of iodine are required for 125 ml of Lugol's solution?   _____

9. A nurse has Chlorpromazine for injection that contains 10 milligrams (mg) per 2 milliliters (ml). He must give a patient 0.025 gram (gm). How many ml should he give the patient? (*Hint:* 1 gm = 1000 mg.)   _____

10. A hemoglobin (hgb) test measures 14.5 grams (gm) of hgb per 100 milliliters (ml) of blood. If the patient has 5.5 quarts (qt) of blood in her body, how many gm of hgb are present? (*Hint:* 1 qt = 1000 ml.)   _____

11. The property tax on a medical center is one mill or $\frac{1}{10}$ of a cent ($0.001) for every $1.00 of appraised value. The medical center has an appraised value of $235,654.00.

    a. What is the tax due for one mill?   _____

    b. What is the tax due if the tax rate is $24\frac{1}{2}$ mills?   _____

12. Time periods for taking X rays are in graduations called impulses. An impulse is a fraction of a second and 30 impulses equal $\frac{1}{2}$ second.

    a. What part of a second is represented by 15 impulses?   _____

    b. How many impulses are required for $1\frac{1}{2}$ seconds?   _____

13. The safe fluoride-to-water ratio is 0.7 to 1.2 parts per million (ppm). What is the range in parts of fluoride that could be added to 200,000 gallons of water? _____

20 Milliliters

AMPICILLIN®
Intramuscular Injections

1 gram per 4 ml

Use the drug label to complete problems 14 to 16.

14. How many total grams (gm) of Ampicillin® are in the vial? _____

15. If a patient is to receive 125 milligrams (mg) of Ampicillin®, how many milliliters (ml) should be injected? (*Hint:* 1 gm = 1000 mg.) _____

16. A patient receives an IM (intramuscular) injection containing $2\frac{1}{2}$ ml of Ampicillin®. How many milligrams did he receive? _____

17. A radiology department has to perform chest X rays on 164 people who had positive skin tests for tuberculosis. Each chest X ray takes 15 minutes.

   a. How many hours will it take to complete all the chest X rays? _____

   b. Three radiologic technologists are working together to take the X rays. During an $8\frac{1}{2}$-hour day, each technician gets two 15-minute breaks and a 30-minute lunch period. How many days will it take the three technologists to complete all the chest X rays? _____

18. An iodine compound used for barium enemas (BE) comes in 8-ounce (oz) concentrated bottles of iodine. This must be diluted to a 25% solution.

   a. What is the total number of oz of solution after the barium is diluted to a 25% solution? _____

   b. How many oz of water should be added to the 8 oz of barium to obtain the correct total amount of solution? _____

   c. If a patient receives a total of 8 oz of the 25% diluted solution, how many oz of concentrated iodine should be used to prepare the 8 oz? _____

Metric and Other Measurements

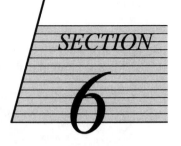

Unit 22 LINEAR MEASUREMENT

BASIC PRINCIPLES OF LINEAR MEASUREMENT

Linear measurement is the measurement of length or distance. In the English system, the units of linear measurement are inches, feet, yards, and miles. In the metric system, the unit for linear measurement is the meter.

The metric system is used in many health care fields. It is easy to use since it is based on units of tens. Units are created by either multiplying or dividing the base unit of measurement by the correct power of ten. Study the other units for the meter and the power of ten they represent in the following chart.

METRIC LINEAR UNIT	SYMBOL	VALUE IN METERS	RELATION TO BASE UNIT
kilometer	km	1,000.0 (10^3)	Multiply by 1,000
hectometer	hm	100.0 (10^2)	Multiply by 100
dekameter	dam	10.0 (10^1)	Multiply by 10
meter	m	1	Base Unit
decimeter	dm	0.1 (10^{-1})	Divide by 10
centimeter	cm	0.01 (10^{-2})	Divide by 100
millimeter	mm	0.001 (10^{-3})	Divide by 1,000

Converting Metric Linear Measurements:

Metrics are easy to convert from unit to unit because they are multiples of ten. Placement of a number in relation to a decimal point represents different powers of ten, so metrics can be converted by moving the decimal point in relationship to the power of ten required.

Example 1: How many meters are in 35.7 kilometers?

First list the measurements in order from largest to smallest.
(*Hint:* A wise teacher once suggested students memorize "**K**ids **h**ave **d**ropped **o**ver **d**ead **c**onverting **m**etrics" to remember the order of k, h, d, o (main unit), d, c, and m.)

km　　hm　　dam　　meters　　dm　　cm　　mm

Movement is three places to the right, so the decimal point is moved three places to the right.

35.7 kilometers = 3 5 . 7 0 0 = 35,700 meters

35.7 km = 35,700 m

Example 2: How many dekameters are in 4,560 millimeters?

First list the measurements in order from largest to smallest.

km　　hm　　dam　　meters　　dm　　cm　　mm

Movement is four places to the left, so the decimal point is moved four places to the left.

4,560 millimeters = 0 4 5 6 0 . 0 = 0.456 dekameter

4,560 mm = 0.456 dam

Converting Metric and English Linear Measurements:

At times it is necessary to convert between metric linear measurements and English linear measurements. Metric linear measurements can be converted to approximate English linear measurements. Common conversion equivalents are shown on the chart.

ENGLISH-METRIC LINEAR EQUIVALENTS				
	1 inch (in)	=	0.0254 meter (m)	
12 inches	= 1 foot (ft)	=	0.3048 meter (m)	
3 feet	= 1 yard (yd)	=	0.9144 meter (m)	
5,280 feet	= 1 mile (mi)	=	1,609 meters (m)	
39.372 inches	= 3.281 feet (ft)	=	1 meter (m)	
	1.094 yards (yd)	=	1 meter (m)	
	0.621 mile (mi)	=	1 kilometer (km)	

The easiest way to convert between English and metric measurements is to set up a proportion.

Example 1:   A group of student nurses is running a 5-kilomter (km) race to raise money for the United Appeal. How many miles (ml) will they run?

1 km = 0.621 mi   Find an English-metric equivalent for this problem

$\dfrac{1 \text{ km}}{0.621 \text{ mi}} \underset{\diagup}{\overset{\diagdown}{=}} \dfrac{5 \text{ km}}{X \text{ mi}}$ Set up a proportion: 1 km : 0.621 mi = 5 km : X mi

$1 \times X = 1\,X$ Multiply the extremes.

$0.621 \times 5 = 3.105$ Multiply the means.

$1X = 3.105$ Write as means equals extremes.

$X = 3.105$ mi   Divide both sides by 1 to find the answer of 3.105 miles.

The students will run 3.105 mi in the 5-km race.

Example 2: A newborn infant measures 22.5 inches (in) at birth. What is the infant's length in centimeters (cm)?

1 in = 0.254 m	Find an English-metric equivalent for this problem.
0. 0 2 54 m = 2.54 cm	Convert meters to centimeters.
$\dfrac{1 \text{ in}}{2.54 \text{ cm}} = \dfrac{22.5 \text{ in}}{X \text{ cm}}$	Set up a proportion: 1 in : 2.54 cm = 22.5 in : X cm
$1 \times X = 1X$	Multiply the extremes.
$2.54 \times 22.5 = 57.15$	Multiply the means.
$1X = 57.15$	Write as means equals extremes.
$X = 57.15$ cm	Divide both sides by 1 to find the answer of 57.15 cm.

The infant measures 22.5 in or 57.15 cm at birth.

PRACTICAL PROBLEMS

1. Convert the following to meters.

   a. 8.45 km _____

   b. 5,689 cm _____

   c. 3,432 dam _____

   d. 54 mm _____

   e. 0.5468 hm _____

2. A public health nurse travels 6,548 m (meters) in one day. How many km (kilometers) does he travel? _____

3. The length of a protozoa is 0.00009712 dam. What is its length in mm (millimeters)? _____

4. An infant is 0.4492 m (meters) long at birth. What is her length in centimeters (cm)? _____

5. A microbiologist measures the length of a bacterium as 0.000163 m and the length of yeast as 0.0087 mm.

   a. Which is longest? (*Hint:* Both must be the same units.) _____

   b. How much longer is the longer specimen than the shorter specimen? _____

6. A heart attack patient starts an exercise program. The first day he walks 0.5 km (kilometers). Each day he increases his distance by 500 m (meters).

   a. At the end of 1 week (7 days), how far is he walking?   _____

   b. How many km does he walk in 1 week?   _____

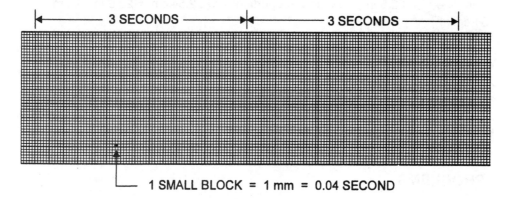

Use the previous figure for problems 7 to 9.

7. One small block on electrocardiograph (ECG) paper is 1 mm wide and represents 0.4 seconds. If a standard ECG runs 12 leads for 6 seconds each, how many mm of paper are required?   _____

8. If a roll of ECG paper contains 9 meters of paper, how many standard ECGs can be run per roll of paper?   _____

9. If rolls of ECG paper cost $436.72 per gross, what is the cost of paper for each standard ECG? (*Hint:* A gross is 12 dozen.)   _____

10. A sterile supply technician can purchase adhesive tape in 50-ft rolls for $14.20. He can also purchase 150-cm rolls of tape for $1.65 each.

    a. Which is the better buy?   _____

    b. What is the difference in price between the large roll and a dozen of the smaller rolls?   _____

11. A newborn infant is 19.5 inches long.

    a. What is her length in meters?   _____

    b. What is her length in centimeters?   _____

12. March of Dimes sponsors a 12-km run. How many miles is the run?   _____

13. A medical lab technologist (MLT) is transferring blood into a sedimentation rate tube that is 4 inches long. To get to the bottom of the tube, should she use an 8-cm or 12-cm pipette? _____

14. A genetic researcher uses 25-meter rolls of chromatography paper at a cost of $47.60 per roll. The paper is cut into 3-inch strips for each test.

   a. How many strips can be obtained per roll? _____

   b. What is the cost of the paper per test? _____

15. A group of patients in a research study are measured and their heights are charted on a graph. What is the average height in centimeters? _____

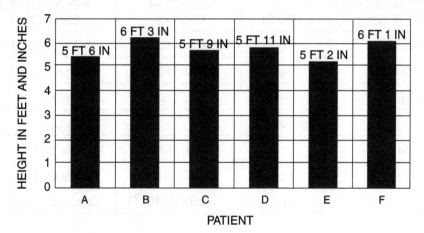

16. A medical office is putting wallpaper border around the upper edge of all of the examining rooms. Two rooms measure 10 feet (ft) 2 inches (in) by 8 ft 3 in, and the other two rooms measure 11 ft 5 in by 9 ft 4 in. The border comes in 6-meter (m) rolls. How many rolls of paper will be needed for the four rooms? (*Hint:* Each room has 4 walls.) _____

Unit 23 **MASS OR WEIGHT MEASUREMENT**

BASIC PRINCIPLES OF MASS OR WEIGHT MEASUREMENT

In the English system, the units for mass or weight measurement are ounces and pounds. In the metric system, the base unit for mass or weight measurement is the gram. Other units for the gram and the power of ten they represent are shown in the following chart.

METRIC MASS OR WEIGHT UNIT	SYMBOL	VALUE IN GRAMS	RELATION TO BASE UNIT
kilogram	kg	1,000.0 (10^3)	Multiply by 1,000
hectogram	hg	100.0 (10^2)	Multiply by 100
dekagram	dag	10.0 (10^1)	Multiply by 10
gram	gm or g	1	Base Unit
decigram	dg	0.1 (10^{-1})	Divide by 10
centigram	cg	0.01 (10^{-2})	Divide by 100
milligram	mg	0.001 (10^{-3})	Divide by 1,000

Converting Metric Mass or Weight Measurements:

Conversion from one unit to another follows the same rules used in working with linear measurement.

Example: How many milligrams are in 0.3467 dekagram?

First list the measurements in order from largest to smallest.

kg　　hg　　dag　　grams　　dg　　cg　　mg

Movement is four places to the right, so the decimal point is moved four places to the right.

0.3467 dekagram = 0 . 3 4 6 7 = 3,467 milligrams

0.3467 dag = 3,467 mg

Converting Metric and English Mass or Weight Measurements:

At times it is necessary to convert between metric mass measurements and English mass measurements. Common conversion equivalent units for converting metric mass or weight units to English units are shown in the following chart.

ENGLISH-METRIC MASS OR WEIGHT EQUIVALENTS

1 ounce (oz) = 0.028 kilogram (kg) or 28 grams (gm)

16 ounces (oz) = 1 pound (lb) = 0.454 kilogram (kg) or 454 grams (gm)

35.27 ounces (oz) = 1 kilogram (kg)

2.2 pounds (lb) = 1 kilogram (kg)

Follow the same rules used for linear measurement to convert English and metric measurements. The easiest way to convert between English and metric measurements is to set up a proportion.

Example: A newborn infant weighs 8 pounds (lb) 6 ounces (oz) at birth. How many kilograms (kg) does he weigh?

8 lb 6 oz = ? oz	First convert the weight to all ounces.
8 × 16 = 128	Multiply 8 lb by 16 (16 oz = 1 lb)
128 + 6 = 134 oz	Add the 6 oz to the 128 oz to find total ounces.
1 oz = 0.028 kg	Find an English-metric equivalent for this problem.
$\dfrac{1 \text{ oz}}{0.028 \text{ kg}} \diagdown\!\!\!=\!\!\!\diagup \dfrac{134 \text{ oz}}{X \text{ kg}}$	Set up a proportion: 1 oz : 0.028 kg = 134 oz : X kg
1 × X = 1X	Multiply the extremes.
0.028 × 134 = 3.752	Multiply the means.
1X = 3.752	Write as means equals extremes.
X = 3.752 kg	Divide both sides by 1 to find the answer of 3.752 kg.

The infant weighs 8 lb 6 oz (134 oz) or 3.752 kg at birth.

PRACTICAL PROBLEMS

1. Convert the following to grams.

   a. 7.563 kg _____

   b. 4,562 mg _____

   c. 56 dag _____

   d. 56.892 cg _____

   e. 0.0921 dg _____

2. A box of cereal weighs 0.448 kilograms (kg). What is its weight in grams (gm)? _____

3. A newborn infant weighs 3,178 grams (gm). What is his weight in kilograms (kg)? _____

4. A patient is to receive 2 grams (gm) of an antibiotic. Tablets available are 500 milligrams (mg). How many tablets should the patient take? _____

5. A patient on a low-salt diet is limited to 1500 mg of sodium (Na) per day. A box of crackers shows 0.320 gram of Na per cracker. How many crackers can the patient eat without exceeding her daily limit of Na? _____

6. A patient is to receive 1.5 grams (gm) of Keflex® per day divided into 3 equal doses.

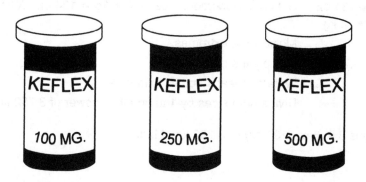

   a. If the above containers of Keflex® capsules are available, which dosage should be used? _____

   b. If the dosage is reduced to 1 gm per day divided into 4 equal doses, what dosage should be used? _____

7. A pathologist weighs 5 tumors and obtains the following weights: 2.2 hg, 520 dg, 34 dag, 420 cg, and 4 mg.

   a. What is the total weight in grams (gm)?   _____

   b. What is the total weight in kilograms (kg)?   _____

   c. What is the average weight of the 5 tumors in milligrams (mg)?   _____

8. If 5 milliliters (ml) of blood contains 5.2 grams (gm) of hemoglobin (hgb), how many kilograms (kg) would be present in 1 quart (qt) of blood? (*Hint:* 1 qt equals 1000 ml.)   _____

9. John weighs 182 pounds (lb). What is his weight in kilograms (kg)?   _____

10. Katy weighs 53.4 kg. What is her weight in lb?   _____

11. A physician orders aminophylline 7.5 mg per kg of body weight. The patient weighs 110 lb.

   a. What dosage of aminophylline should the patient receive?   _____

   b. If aminophylline is available in 0.125-gm tablets, how many tablets should the patient receive?   _____

12. A weight loss clinic graphs the weights of 5 patients.

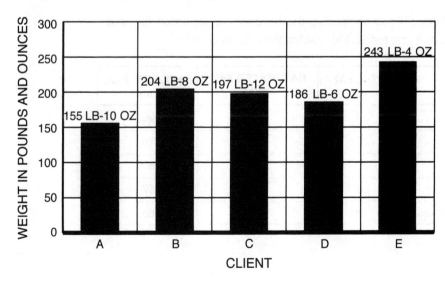

   a. What is the total weight of the patients in kg? (*Hint:* One pound equals 16 ounces.)   _____

   b. What is the average weight of the 5 patients in kg?   _____

13. A label on snack crackers shows a total of 6,000 mg of fat including 1.5 gm of saturated fat. What percent of the total fat is saturated fat?   _____

14. A lab technician is preparing agar medium. The medium requires 21 grams (gm) of agar, 500 mg of dextrose, 3 dg of sodium, and 1 cg of potassium per 1000 milliliters (ml) of distilled water.

    a. What is the total weight in gm of the dry ingredients?   _____

    b. If each culture dish uses 50 ml of the agar medium, what would the total weight in mg of dry ingredients be per culture dish?   _____

15. A patient weighs 55 pounds (lb) and 12 ounces (oz). Meperidine hydrochloride is ordered for pain at a dosage of 6 milligrams (mg) per kilogram (kg) of body weight in a 24-hour period. Meperidine hydrochloride is available in injection form with 50 mg per ml.

    a. What is the patient's weight in kg?   _____

    b. What dosage in mg of meperidine hydrochloride should be given to the patient q4h (every four hours)? (*Hint:* This is per dosage, not the 24-hour dosage.)   _____

    c. How many ml of meperidine hydrochloride would the patient be able to receive in a 24-hour period?   _____

16. A registered dietitian (RD) is comparing the fat content, saturated fat, and cholesterol in different fast foods. He creates the following chart.

FAST FOOD	TOTAL FAT gm	SATURATED FAT dag	CHOLESTEROL mg
Whopper	39	110	90
Big Mac	26	93	76
Pan Pizza	30	120	60
Italian Sub	25	90	57
Taco Salad with Salsa	56	163	65

a. Which fast food has the highest percent of saturated fat compared to total fat content? _____

b. Which fast food has the highest percent of cholesterol compared to total fat content? _____

c. If the dietitian wants to recommend the fast food that has the lowest average percent of saturated fat and cholesterol compared to total fat, which food should he recommend? _____

Unit 24 VOLUME OR LIQUID MEASUREMENT

BASIC PRINCIPLES OF VOLUME OR LIQUID MEASUREMENT

In the English system, the units for volume or liquid measurement are drops, teaspoons, tablespoons, ounces, pints, and quarts. In the metric system, the base unit for volume or liquid measurement is the liter. Other units for the liter and the power of ten they represent are shown in the following chart.

METRIC LIQUID OR VOLUME UNIT	SYMBOL	VALUE IN LITERS	RELATION TO BASE UNIT
kiloliter	kl	1,000.0 (10^3)	Multiply by 1,000
hectoliter	hl	100.0 (10^2)	Multiply by 100
dekaliter	dal	10.0 (10^1)	Multiply by 10
liter	l	1	Base Unit
deciliter	dl	0.1 (10^{-1})	Divide by 10
centiliter	cl	0.01 (10^{-2})	Divide by 100
milliliter	ml	0.001 (10^{-3})	Divide by 1,000

Note: The chart shows milliliters, but it is important to remember that 1 milliliter (ml) is the same as 1 cubic centimeter (cc). In many health fields, cubic centimeters (cc) are used in place of milliliters (ml). Therefore remember that *1 ml = 1 cc.*

Converting Metric Volume Measurements:

Conversion from one unit to another follows the same rules used in working with linear or mass measurement.

Example: How many hectoliters (hl) are in 56,973 centiliters (cl)?

First list the measurements in order from largest to smallest.

kl   hl   dal   liter   dl   cl   ml

Movement is four places to the left, so the decimal point is moved four places to the left.

56,973 centiliters = 5 6 9 7 3 . 0 = 5.6973 hectoliters

56,973 cl = 5.673 hl

Converting Metric and English Volume or Liquid Measurements:

At times it is necessary to convert between metric volume measurements and English volume measurements. Common conversion equivalent units used to convert English and metric volume or liquid measurements are shown on the chart.

ENGLISH-METRIC VOLUME OR LIQUID EQUIVALENTS				
		1 drop (gtt)	=	0.0667 milliliter (ml)
		15 drops (gtt)	=	1.0 milliliter (ml)
		1 teaspoon (tsp)	=	5.0 milliliters (ml)
3 teaspoons	=	1 tablespoon (tbsp)	=	15.0 milliliters (ml)
		1 ounce (oz)	=	30.0 milliliters (ml)
8 ounces (oz)	=	1 cup (cp)	=	240.0 milliliters (ml)
2 cups (cp)	=	1 pint (pt)	=	500.0 milliliters (ml)
2 pints (pt)	=	1 quart (qt)	=	1000.0 milliliters (ml)

Follow the same rules used for linear or mass and weight measurements to convert between English and metric units. The easiest way to convert between English and metric measurements is to set up a proportion.

Example: A patient on an I & O (Intake and Output) record drinks 2½ cups (cp) of coffee. The geriatric assistant must record this amount in cubic centimeters (cc). How many cc does he record on the I & O record?

2½ cp = 2.5 cp	First convert the fraction to a decimal fraction.
1 cp = 240 cc	Find an English-metric equivalent for this problem. (*Hint:* Remember 1 ml = 1 cc.)
$\dfrac{1 \text{ cp}}{240 \text{ cc}} = \dfrac{2.5 \text{ cp}}{X \text{ cc}}$	Set up a proportion: 1 cp : 240 cc = 2.5 cp : X cc
1 × X = 1X	Multiply the extremes.
240 × 2.5 = 600	Multiply the means.
1X = 600	Write as means equals extremes.
X = 600 cc	Divide both sides by 1 to find the answer of 600 cc.

The patient drank 2½ cp or 600 cc of coffee.

PRACTICAL PROBLEMS

1. Convert the following to liters.

    a. 569.23 cl   _____

    b. 351.6 hl   _____

    c. 88.2 dl   _____

    d. 91.07 kl   _____

    e. 0.5185 dal   _____

2. A patient is told to force fluids to 3 liters (l) per day. How many milliliters (ml) should she drink?   _____

3. Prepared infant formula comes in 1-liter (l) cans. If an infant drinks 150 ml per feeding, how many feedings are in 1 can of formula?   _____

4. During a 24-hour period, a patient receives 2.5 liters (l) of intravenous (IV) solution and drinks 2,440 cubic centimeters (cc) of fluids. In the same period, he urinates or voids 3,100 cc of urine. (*Hint:* Remember 1 ml = 1 cc.)

    a. What is his total intake of IV solution and fluids in l?   _____

    b. How much more total intake did he have in cc than his total urine output?   _____

5. A beaker of diluting solution holds 1½ quarts (qt). Each blood test uses 3 centiliters (cl) of diluting solution. How many blood tests can be performed with the full beaker of solution?   _____

6. A patient is on an Intake and Output (I & O) record. During one day she drinks 2 juice glasses of juice, $3\frac{1}{2}$ water glasses of water, $3\frac{1}{4}$ cups of coffee, and $1\frac{3}{4}$ large bowls of broth.

CONTAINER	CONTENTS IN cc
Juice Glass	120 cc
Water Glass	180 cc
Large Glass	240 cc
Small Bowl	100 cc
Large Bowl	200 cc
Cup	180 cc
Coffee Pot	360 cc

   a. Using the conversions shown in the chart, calculate her total oral intake in cubic centimeters (cc).   _____

   b. If she must have .002 kiloliter (kl) of fluid per day, how many more cc of fluid must she drink? (*Hint:* Remember 1 cc = 1 ml.)   _____

7. A serum is being given to a patient to desensitize the patient for a variety of allergies. Each week the dosage is increased by .01 centiliters (cl). If the patient receives 0.5 milliliters (ml) the first week, what dosage would he receive the 6th week?   _____

8. To perform a Gram's stain on a bacteria slide, a technician uses 5 ml of gentian violet, 8 ml of Gram's iodine, 1.4 cl of acetone-alcohol, 1.0 cl of safranin, and 0.05 liters (l) of distilled water. How many l of solutions and distilled water would she need to perform 150 tests?   _____

9. Principen® suspension is available as shown.

> **200 Milliliters**
>
> ## *PRINCIPEN® SUSPENSION*
> ### *Ampicillin U.S.P.*
>
> **250 milligrams in 5 milliliters**

    a. How many mg are in 1 ml of suspension?   _____

    b. If a patient receives 2 ml q6h (every 6 hours), how many mg will he receive in a 24-hour period?   _____

10. A prepared enema contains 6 ounces (oz) of solution. How many ml of solution are in the enema?   _____

11. Most adults have 5,000 to 6,000 ml of blood in their bodies. How many quarts (qt) of blood do they have?   _____

12. A child receives 2 teaspoons (tsp) of a penicillin suspension q6h (every six hours). The label states that there are 125 mg of penicillin in 5 ml.

    a. How many ml of suspension would he receive in a 24-hour period?   _____

    b. How many gm of penicillin would he receive in 24 hours?   _____

13. To stain a blood slide, a technician uses 10 drops (gtt) of Wright's stain, 10 gtt of buffer solution, and 40 gtt of distilled water.

    a. If she stains 9 blood smear slides, how many ml of stain, buffer solution, and distilled water does she use?   _____

    b. If she stains 17 blood smear slides, how many teaspoons (tsp) of stain, buffer solution, and distilled water does she use?   _____

14. A pharmacist is filling a prescription for triazolam, a sedative, for a patient with insomnia. The label provides the following information.

> 100 Tablets
> 6506-01-220-5833
>
> **Triazolam Tablets, USP**
>
> 0.125 mg
>
> Caution: Federal law prohibits dispensing without prescription.

a. If the patient is to take 0.5 mg HS qd (at bedtime every day), how many tablets will he take each night? _____

b. The pharmacist must fill the prescription for a one-week supply. How many tablets should she dispense to the patient? _____

15. To prepare a vaginal irrigation, a nurse must use 3 teaspoons (tsp) of vinegar and 1.5 liters (l) of water.

a. How many ml of vinegar should she use? _____

b. How many quarts (qt) of water should she use? _____

c. If she prepares a solution using only 500 ml of water, how many ml of vinegar should she use? _____

16. A patient drinks 1½ quarts (qt) of water, 3 cups (cp) of coffee, 12 tablespoons of broth (tbsp), ¾ pint (pt) of milk, and 12 ounces (oz) of juice. What is his total intake in liters (l)? _____

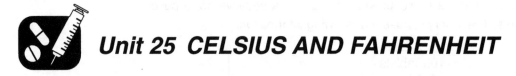

Unit 25 CELSIUS AND FAHRENHEIT

BASIC PRINCIPLES OF CELSIUS AND FAHRENHEIT CONVERSIONS

The temperature measurement used most commonly in the United States is the Fahrenheit (F) scale. In the metric system used by most other countries, Celsius (C) or Centigrade is the measurement used. A comparison of the two systems is shown on the diagram.

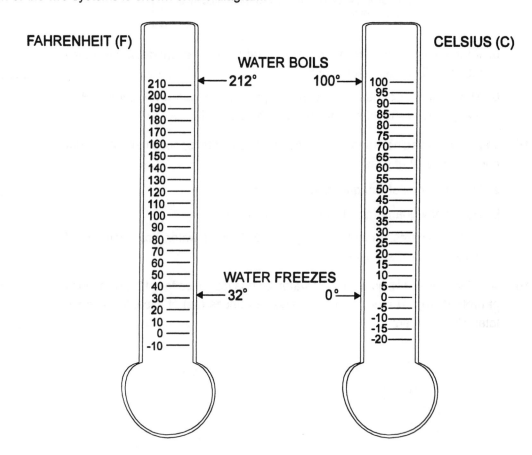

In the Fahrenheit system, the freezing point is 32° and the boiling point is 212°. In the Celsius system, the freezing point is 0° and the boiling point is 100°.

Converting Fahrenheit to Celsius:

To convert Fahrenheit temperatures to Celsius temperatures, the following formula is used:

$$C = (F - 32) \times \tfrac{5}{9} \qquad or \qquad C = (F - 32) \times 0.5556$$

Example: Convert 80°F to degrees Celsius.

$$C = (80 - 32) \times \tfrac{5}{9} \qquad or \qquad C = (80 - 32) \times 0.5556$$

$$C = 48 \times \tfrac{5}{9} \qquad or \qquad C = 48 \times 0.5556$$

$$C = 26\tfrac{2}{3} \text{ or } 26.7° \qquad or \qquad C = 26.6688 \text{ or } 26.7°$$

Converting Celsius to Fahrenheit:

To convert Celsius temperatures to Fahrenheit temperatures, the following formula is used:

$$F = \tfrac{9}{5} C + 32 \qquad or \qquad F = 1.8 C + 32$$

Example: Convert 60°C to degrees Fahrenheit.

$$F = \tfrac{9}{5} \times 60 + 32 \qquad or \qquad F = 1.8 \times 60 + 32$$

$$F = 108 + 32 \qquad or \qquad F = 108 + 32$$

$$F = 140° \qquad or \qquad F = 140°$$

PRACTICAL PROBLEMS

Convert the following temperatures to degrees Celsius (°C):

1. 59°F   _____

2. 131°F   _____

3. 40°F   _____

4. 180.8°F   _____

5. 82.4°F   _____

Convert the following temperatures to degrees Fahrenheit (°F):

6. 70°C   _____

7. 10°C   _____

8. 32°C   _____

9. 48.7°C   _____

10. 18.25°C   _____

11. The normal oral body temperature is 37°C. What is the normal oral body
     temperature in °F?   _____

12. The normal range for body temperature is 97° to 100°F. What is the normal
     range for body temperature in °C?   _____

13. A home health aide is preparing a warm-water bottle for his patient. The order
     states the temperature should be 46.1°C. The only thermometer in the home
     has a Fahrenheit scale. What °F temperature should he use? _____

14. A physical therapist (PT) is filling a whirlpool bath after it has been
     disinfected. The temperature of the bath should be set at 100°F. The digital
     control on the whirlpool bath is calculated for degrees Celsius. What °C
     temperature should she use?   _____

15. A patient care technician (PCT) has an order to apply an aquamatic pad to a
     patient's leg for 20 minutes at a temperature of 35°C. The control on the
     aquamatic unit is calculated in degrees F. What °F should he use? _____

16. A surgical nurse is teaching a patient how to fill a portable sitz bath for the
     patient to use after rectal surgery. The sitz tub unit is filled with water at
     40.6°C and the bag of water to refill the tub is filled with water at 48.9°C. The
     patient only has a Fahrenheit scale thermometer at home.

     a. What temperature should be used in °F for the sitz tub? _____

     b. What temperature should be used in °F for the sitz bag? _____

17. A liver has been removed from a brain-dead donor for transplant. During the helicopter flight to deliver the liver, it must be kept at 36.5°F. What is the temperature in °C?

         _____

18. A patient is admitted to a burn unit with second- and third-degree burns over 65% of his body. The EMT who rescued the patient from his burning apartment states that the firefighters estimated the temperature of the fire to be between 250° to 275°C. What is the range in °F?

         _____

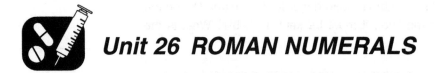

Unit 26 ROMAN NUMERALS

BASIC PRINCIPLES OF ROMAN NUMERALS

Roman numerals are used in health care for some drugs and solutions. At times, they are used while ordering supplies. Roman numerals use letters or symbols to represent numbers. The common equivalent values between Arabic numbers and Roman numerals are shown on the chart.

ARABIC	ROMAN	ARABIC	ROMAN	ARABIC	ROMAN
1	I	8	VIII	60	LX
2	II	9	IX	70	LXX
3	III	10	X	80	LXXX
4	IV	20	XX	90	XC
5	V	30	XXX	100	C
6	VI	40	XL	500	D
7	VII	50	L	1000	M

The key symbols are the I, V, X, L, C, D, and M. By using these symbols, any number can be formed. Usually no more than three of any one symbol is used to represent a number. If a letter or symbol is repeated in sequence, the numbers are added. For example, III is 1 + 1 + 1 or 3. If a symbol for a smaller number is used after the symbol for a larger number, all of the numbers are added together. For example, LXVI is 50 + 10 + 5 + 1 or 66. If a symbol for a smaller number is used in front of the symbol for a larger number, the smaller number is subtracted from the larger number. For example, XC is equal to 100 − 10 or 90.

Example: Convert 134 to Roman numerals.

100 = C   30 = XXX   4 = 5 − 1 = IV

134 = CXXXIV

Example: Convert CDXXIX to Arabic numbers.

CD = 500 − 100 = 400

XX = 10 + 10 = 20

IX = 10 − 1 = 9

CDXXIX = 400 + 20 + 9 = 429

PRACTICAL PROBLEMS

Convert the following Arabic numbers to Roman numerals:

1. 27 _____

2. 368 _____

3. 94 _____

4. 749 _____

5. 2648 _____

Convert the following Roman numerals to Arabic numbers:

6. XXIII _____

7. LXXXVI _____

8. CCXIX _____

9. MCMXCIV _____

10. DCCCXCVIII _____

11. A child is to receive grains (gr) X of aspirin. Aspirin is available in gr V tablets. How many tablets should the child receive? _____

12. Copy paper is available in reams of D sheets. A medical office orders MMD pages. How many reams of paper are ordered? _____

13. The cornerstone of a hospital shows the date when the hospital was built as MCMXLVII. When was the hospital built? _____

14. A registered nurse (RN) is evaluating an order for pain medication for a patient. The patient is to receive gr (grain) I of codeine q4h (every four hours) IM (intramuscular). The nurse knows that the total dosage in a 24-hour period should not exceed gr VI.

> 30 ml Multiple Dose Vial
> 3406-07-165-4160
>
> **Codeine Sulfate**
>
> Gr V / 10 ml
>
> Caution: Federal law prohibits dispensing without prescription.

a. How many ml of codeine should be injected for gr I?   _____

b. If the patient receives this dose q4h, will this exceed the maximum dose allowed per 24-hour period?   _____

15. A medical assistant does an inventory of file folders and counts CCLX beige folders, CDXLVI yellow folders, CCCXXXIX blue folders, and MCMLXXXIII white folders.

a. What is the total number of file folders in Roman numerals?   _____

b. What is the total number of file folders in Arabic numbers?   _____

16. A patient is to receive a total of grains (gr) XL of acetaminophen every 24 hours. He gets the medication every 6 hours.

a. What is the dosage every 6 hours in Roman numerals?   _____

b. If acetaminophen is available in gr V capsules, how many capsules does he receive every 6 hours?   _____

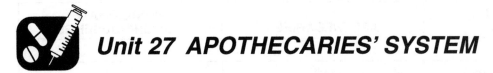# *Unit 27* **APOTHECARIES' SYSTEM**

BASIC PRINCIPLES OF THE APOTHECARIES' SYSTEM

The apothecaries' system is an old English system of measurement. Even though it is being replaced by the metric system, it is still used for certain medications. In the apothecaries' system, the basic unit of weight is the grain. The basic units for volume or liquid measurement are the minim, fluid dram, and fluid ounce.

These unit abbreviations are usually written in front of the number. Approximate equivalent values are shown in the chart on page 154.

Frequently Roman numerals are used in the apothecary system. In addition, symbols are used for dram and ounce as shown on the chart. The symbol for ounce (℥) has one more loop than the symbol for dram (ʒ). It is important to learn the symbols since a serious medication error can result if the wrong amount is used. Another abbreviation that is used frequently in the apothecaries' system is *ss* which stands for one-half. In addition, as mentioned previously, the abbreviations or symbols for the apothecary system are usually written before the quantity. The following chart shows some examples of apothecaries' abbreviations and their interpretation.

APOTHECARY	INTERPRETATION	APOTHECARY	INTERPRETATION
gr I	one grain	gr 1/5	one-fifth grain
gr vi	six grains	℥ iiss	two and one-half ounces
gr ss	one-half grain	℥ 1/4	one quarter ounce
gr iss	one and one-half grains	ʒ iss	one and one-half drams

APPROXIMATE METRIC	APOTHECARIES'	APPROXIMATE ENGLISH/HOUSEHOLD
Dry		
0.25 milligram (mg)	$\frac{1}{250}$ grain (gr)	
0.5 milligram (mg)	$\frac{1}{120}$ grain (gr)	
1 milligram (mg)	$\frac{1}{60}$ grain (gr)	
2 milligrams (mg)	$\frac{1}{30}$ grain (gr)	
4 milligrams (mg)	$\frac{1}{15}$ grain (gr)	
10 milligrams (mg)	$\frac{1}{6}$ grain (gr)	
15 milligrams (mg)	$\frac{1}{4}$ grain (gr)	
30 milligrams (mg)	$\frac{1}{2}$ grain (gr)	
45 milligrams (mg)	$\frac{3}{4}$ grain (gr)	
60 milligrams (mg)	1 grain (gr)	
100 milligrams (mg)	$1\frac{1}{2}$ grain (gr)	
500 milligrams (mg)	$7\frac{1}{2}$ grains (gr)	$\frac{1}{8}$ teaspoon (tsp)
1 gram (gm)	15 grains (gr)	$\frac{1}{4}$ teaspoon (tsp)
4 grams (gm)	1 dram (ʒ or dr) or 60 grains (gr)	1 teaspoon (tsp)
15 grams (gm)	4 drams (ʒ IV)	1 tablespoon (tbsp)
30 grams (gm)	8 drams (ʒ VIII) or 1 ounce (ʒ)	2 tablespoons (tbsp) or 1 ounce (oz)
360 grams (gm)	12 ounces (ʒ XII) or 1 pound (lb)	16 ounces (oz) or 1 pound (lb)
1 kilogram (kg)		2.2 pounds (lb)
Volume or Liquid		
0.06 milliliter (ml)	1 minim (m)	1 drop (gtt)
1 milliliter (ml)	15 minims (m)	15 drops (gtt)
4–5 milliliters (ml)	60 minims (m) or 1 dram (ʒ)	60–75 drops (gtt) or 1 teaspoon (tsp)
15 milliliters (ml)	4 drams (ʒ IV)	1 tablespoon (tbsp)
30 milliliters (ml)	8 drams (ʒ VIII) or 1 ounce (ʒ)	2 tablespoons (tbsp) or 1 ounce (oz)
500 milliliters (ml)	16 ounces (ʒ XVI) or 1 pint (pt)	16 ounces (oz) or 1 pint (pt)
1000 milliliters (ml)	2 pints (pt) or 1 quart (qt)	2 pints (pt) or 1 quart (qt)

Converting Units in the Apothecaries' System:

To convert units in the apothecaries' system, find equivalent measurements on the chart and set up a proportion.

Example 1: How many grains (gr) are in 6 drams (dr)?

1 dr = 60 gr	Find an equivalent for this problem.
$\dfrac{1 \text{ dr}}{60 \text{ gr}} \diagdown \!\!\!= \!\!\!\diagup \dfrac{6 \text{ dr}}{X \text{ gr}}$	Set up a proportion: 1 gr : 60 gr = 6 dr : X gr
$1 \times X = 1X$	Multiply the extremes.
$60 \times 6 = 360$	Multiply the means.
$1X = 360$	Write as means equals extremes.
$X = 360$ gr	Divide both sides by 1 to find the answer of 360 grains.

There are 360 grains in 6 drams.

Example 2: How many drams (dr) are in 240 minims (m)?

1 dr = 60 m	Find an equivalent for this problem.
$\dfrac{1 \text{ dr}}{60 \text{ m}} \diagdown \!\!\!= \!\!\!\diagup \dfrac{X \text{ dr}}{240}$	Set up a proportion: 1 dr : 60 m = X dr : 240 m
$1 \times 240 = 240$	Multiply the extremes.
$60 \times X = 60X$	Multiply the means.
$60X = 240$	Write as means equals extremes.
$X = 4$ dr	Divide both sides by 60 to find the answer of 4 drams.

There are 4 drams in 240 minims.

Converting Apothecary and Metric or English Measurements:

To convert units between the three systems, use the values shown on the chart to set up a proportion. It is important to note that these are approximate equivalent values. Exact values are not obtained when converting between systems of measurement.

Example 1: A medical laboratory technician is preparing a solution. She needs 20 grams (gr) of baking soda for the solution. The only scale weighs in grains (gr). How may grains of baking soda should she use?

1 gram = 15 grains   Find an apothecary-metric equivalent for this problem.

$$\frac{1 \text{ gm}}{15 \text{ gr}} \diagdown \!\!\!\!\! = \!\!\!\!\! \diagup \frac{20 \text{ gm}}{X \text{ gr}}$$ Set up a proportion: 1 gm : 15 gr = 20 gm : X gr

$1 \times X = 1X$ Multiply the extremes.

$15 \times 20 = 300$ Multiply the means.

$1X = 300$ Write as means equals extremes.

$X = 300 \text{gr}$ Divide both sides by 1 to find the answer of 300 grains.

She needs 300 grains or 20 grams of baking soda for the solution.

Example 2: The medical laboratory technician also needs 90 minims (m) of normal saline for the solution. Her graduate measures in milliliters (ml) or cubic centimeters (cc). She knows 1 ml equals 1 cc. How many ml or cc or normal saline should she use?

1 ml = 15 m   Find an apothecary-metric equivalent for this problem.

$$\frac{1 \text{ ml}}{15 \text{m}} \diagdown \!\!\!\!\! = \!\!\!\!\! \diagup \frac{X \text{ ml}}{90 \text{ m}}$$ Set up a proportion: 1 ml: 15 m = X ml : 90 m

$1 \times 90 = 90$ Multiply the extremes.

$15 \times X = 15\ X$ Multiply the means.

$15X = 90$ Write as means equals extremes.

$X = 6 \text{ ml}$ Divide both sides by 15 to find the answer of 6 ml.

She needs 90 minims or 6 ml of normal saline for the solution.

PRACTICAL PROBLEMS

1.   Convert the following units as indicated:

    a. 21 grains to grams   _____

    b. 90 milliliters to minims   _____

    c. 32 drams to tablespoons   _____

    d. 9 tablespoons to minims   _____

    e. 3 milliliters to drops   _____

    f. 0.2 gram to grains   _____

    g. $\frac{1}{8}$ grain to grams   _____

    h. ss ounce to minims   _____

2. A child must take gr XXX of acetaminophen. How many teaspoons (tsp) should she take? (*Hint:* Review Roman numerals.)   _____

Use the diagram to fill in the values indicated by the (?) shown for problems 3 to 6.

3. _____

4. _____

5. _____

6. _____

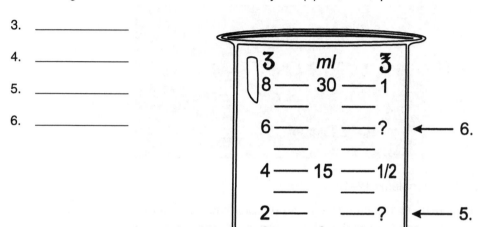

7. A bottle of blood staining solution contains 40 drams (dr).

    a. How many milliliters (ml) does it contain?   _____

    b. How many ounces (oz) does it contain?   _____

8. A patient can take 1 teaspoon (tsp) of cough medicine q4h (every 4 hours).

    a. How many drams (dr) of cough medicine can he take in 24 hours?   _____

    b. How many milliliters (ml) of cough medicine can he take in 24 hours?   _____

9. A cancer patient is given gr ¼ of morphine sulfate q4h (every 4 hours). How many mg of morphine does she receive in a 24-hour period?   _____

10. A nurse must give a patient gr 7½ of aminophylline. Tablets available are 250 mg. How many tablets should the nurse give the patient?   _____

11. A patient with angina uses nitroglycerine sublingually (SL) (under the tongue) for chest pain. The patient has 0.2-mg tablets and must take gr $\frac{1}{150}$. How many tablets should she take?   _____

---

20 Milliliters

SECONAL® SODIUM
Secobarbital Sodium

50 mg (gr $\frac{3}{4}$) per ml

Use the previous diagram for problems 12–14.

12. Using the equivalent value of 1 grain (gr) equals 60 milligrams (mg), what is the difference in mg between the solution shown and the normal equivalent value?   _____

13. If a patient is to receive 100 mg of Seconal®, how many ml should be given to the patient?   _____

14. A patient receives 1$\frac{1}{2}$ ml of Seconal®.

    a. According to the label shown, how many mg of Seconal® does the patient receive?   _____

    b. According to the label shown, how many gr of Seconal® will the patient receive?   _____

15. Sulfasuxidine tablets are available in gr VIIss. A patient is told to take 2.0 gm (grams). How many tablets should she take? (*Hint:* ss equals $\frac{1}{2}$.)   _____

16. A patient is told to take 2000 mg of Donnatol® liquid. The bottle is labeled "Ʒ I equals gr XV." How many teaspoons should the patient take?   _____

17. A bottle of elixir of phenobarbital is labeled gr XV per ml. An infant is to receive 500 mg.

    a. How many ml should the infant receive?   _____

    b. How many minims should the infant receive?   _____

18. If an infant is given 5 drops (gtt) of elixir of phenobarbital labeled 300 mg per ml, how many grains (gr) of phenobarbital does the infant receive?   _____

Measurement Instruments

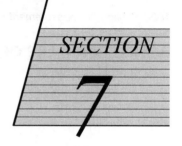

Unit 28 RULERS OR TAPE MEASURES

BASIC PRINCIPLES OF READING RULERS OR TAPE MEASURES

A ruler is a measuring device. Two types of rulers used in health occupations are a tape measure, used to measure the height of infants, and a height beam on a scale, used to measure the height of children and adults.

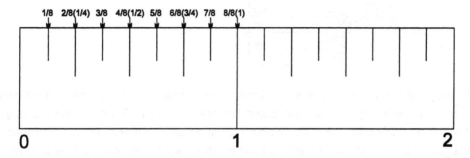

Most tape measures are divided into inches and fractions of inches. In the tape measure shown, each small line represents $\frac{1}{8}$ of an inch (in). Note that fractions are reduced to lowest terms. For example, $\frac{2}{8} = \frac{1}{4}$ after both the 2 and 4 are divided by 2. The long lines represent inches and are marked by a number such as the 1 or 2.

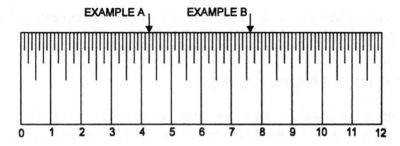

Example A: The reading is 2 lines past 4 inches (in). Since each small line is $\frac{1}{8}$ in, this would be $4\frac{2}{8}$ or $4\frac{1}{4}$ in.

Example B: This reading is 5 lines past 7 inches (in). Since each small line is $\frac{1}{8}$ in, this would be $7\frac{5}{8}$ in.

BASIC PRINCIPLES OF READING HEIGHT BARS

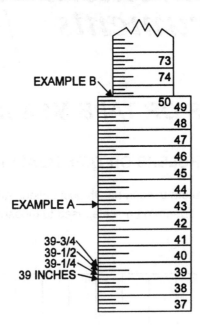

The height bar on a scale is also marked in inches and fractions of inches. On the bar shown, each small line represents $\frac{1}{4}$ of an inch. Each large line is marked and represents an inch. To accommodate varying heights the top part of the bar separates from the bottom part at an area called a "break." To measure height measurements less than 50 inches, the bar is read in an upward direction. To measure height measurements above 50 inches, measurements are read in a downward direction and recorded directly at the break in the scale.

Example A: The reading is below 50 inches so the scale is read in an upward direction. Since it is two lines above the 43, the reading is $43\frac{2}{4}$ or $43\frac{1}{2}$ in.

Example B: The reading is above 50 inches so the scale is read in a downward direction at the break. Since this is 3 lines below the 74, the reading is $74\frac{3}{4}$ in.

CONVERTING INCHES TO FEET AND INCHES

Since a person's height is not stated as $74\frac{3}{4}$ in, the inches must be converted to feet and inches. There are 12 inches (in) in 1 foot (ft), so the inches are divided by 12. The remainder is left in inches.

Example: Convert 74¾ inches to feet (ft) and inches (in).

$$
\begin{array}{r}
6 \text{ ft} \\
12 \overline{)7\ 4\ \tfrac{3}{4}} \\
7\ 2 \\
\hline
2\ \tfrac{3}{4} \text{ remainder} = \text{in}
\end{array}
$$

74¾ in = 6 ft 2¾ in

PRACTICAL PROBLEMS

Use the diagram for problems 1 to 6. Write the correct measurement indicated by the number.

1. _____
2. _____
3. _____
4. _____
5. _____
6. _____

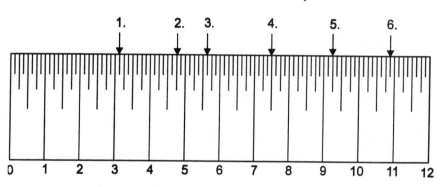

Use the diagram for problems 7 to 10. Write the measurement in inches (in).

7. _____
8. _____
9. _____
10. _____

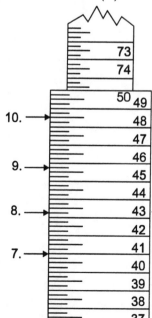

Use the diagram for problems 11 to 14. Read the measurement at the break and record in inches (in).

11. _____

12. _____

13. _____

14. _____

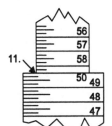
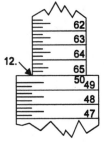
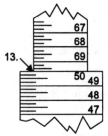
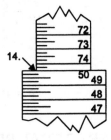

Convert the following inches to feet (ft) and inches (in).

15.   38 in   _____

16.   47¼ in   _____

17.   53½ in   _____

18.   58¼ in   _____

19.   67¾ in   _____

20.   74½ in   _____

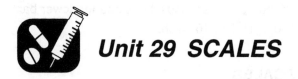 *Unit 29 SCALES*

BASIC PRINCIPLES OF READING SCALES

Scales are used in many health occupations. Examples include scales used in pharmacies to weigh medications, dietary departments to weigh food, and dental laboratories to weigh dental materials. Most of the newer scales are digital or electronic. They are easy to read because the weight is displayed in numbers on the screen, similar to the way the numbers appear on a calculator screen. However, many health care facilities still use scales that must be balanced to obtain the weight.

Two very common scales are beam-balance scales and infant scales. The beam-balance scale usually consists of two weight bars.

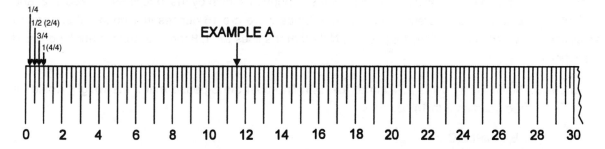

This is the top weight bar. It measures pounds and fractions of pounds up to 50 pounds. Each small line represents ¼ pound (lb). Note that the long lines for odd-numbered pounds such as 1 and 3 are not marked.

Example A: Since this is two lines past the 11-pound mark, the weight would be 11²⁄4 or 11½ lb.

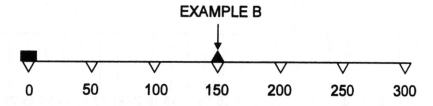

This is the bottom weight bar. It measures weight in 50-pound increments. For an adult who weighs more than 50 pounds, the lower weight bar is adjusted first. The weight is moved until the scale balance bar drops down to show that the weight is too heavy. Then the weight is moved back one 50-pound increment and the top weight bar is adjusted until the balance bar swings freely and shows accurate weight. The weight on the bottom bar is then added to the weight on the top bar to obtain the correct reading.

Example B: The bottom weight is set at 150 pounds. If the upper bar reads 11½, and the lower bar reads 150, the patient's weight would be 150 + 11½ or 161½ lb.

BASIC PRINCIPLES OF READING INFANT SCALES

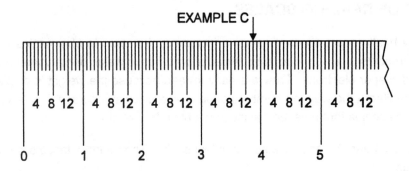

Infant scales vary. The scale shown has increments of pounds shown by the long lines marked 1, 2, and so forth. The smaller lines represent ounces (oz). Since there are 16 ounces in 1 pound, there are 15 small lines between the long lines for pounds. Note that the lines for 4, 8, and 12 ounces are longer and are labeled.

Example C: Since the arrow is pointing at the 14th line past the 3-pound mark, the weight would be recorded as 3 lb 14 oz.

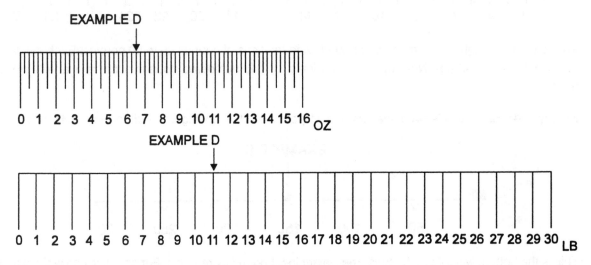

This infant scale has a lower weight bar to measure pounds. The upper weight bar measures ounces and fractions of ounces. Each large line represents one ounce. Each small line represents ¼ of an ounce.

Example D: The lower weight bar is set at 11 pounds (lb). The upper weight bar is at the second line past the 6-ounce (oz) mark and represents $6\frac{2}{4}$ or $6\frac{1}{2}$ oz. The correct weight reading would be 11 lb and $6\frac{1}{2}$ oz.

PRACTICAL PROBLEMS

Use the diagram for problems 1 to 5. Write the correct weight indicated by the numbers above the scale. (*Hint:* Remember to add the weight on the lower bar to the weight on the top bar.)

1. _____

2. _____

3. _____

4. _____

5. _____

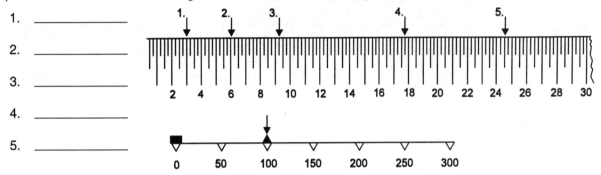

Use the diagram to complete problems 6 to 10. Write the correct weight indicated by the numbers above the scale.

6. _____

7. _____

8. _____

9. _____

10. _____

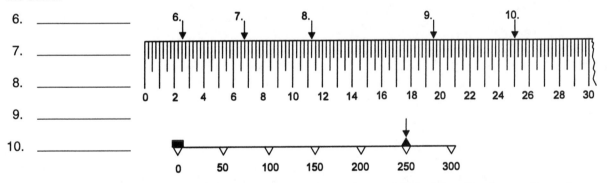

Use the diagram to complete problems 11 to 15. Write the correct weight indicated by the numbers above the scale.

11. _____

12. _____

13. _____

14. _____

15. _____

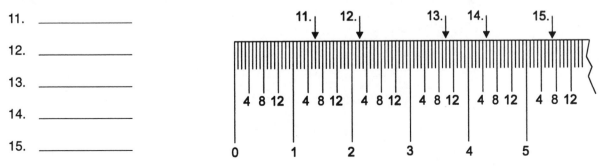

Use the diagram to complete problems 16 to 20. Write the correct weight indicated by the numbers above the scale. (*Hint:* Remember that this scale has two bars that must be read and added together.)

16. _____

17. _____

18. _____

19. _____

20. _____

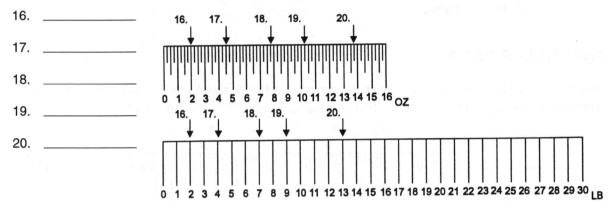

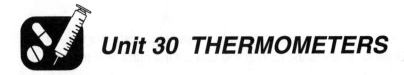

Unit 30 THERMOMETERS

BASIC PRINCIPLES OF READING THERMOMETERS

Thermometers are used in many health occupations. A major use is to record body temperature. Many thermometers are electronic or digital. They are easy to read because the body temperature appears on a screen, similar to the way numbers appear on a calculator screen. However, some thermometers are not electronic.

A common example is the clinical thermometer. This consists of a column of mercury or alcohol inside a glass stem. Body heat causes the mercury or alcohol to expand and move up the stem so the temperature can be recorded.

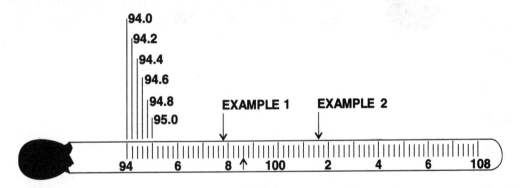

The previous diagram is a clinical thermometer with a Fahrenheit scale of measurement. Each long line represents one degree. Usually only even numbers are marked on the thermometer. Long lines for odd-numbered degrees are not marked. On some thermometers there is an arrow or long line by 98.6°F (degrees Fahrenheit) which is the normal oral body temperature. Each small line represents 0.2 (two-tenths) degree. The temperature is recorded to the nearest two-tenths of a degree.

Example 1: The arrow is on the fourth line past the long line indicating 97 degrees. The reading is 97.8°F.

Example 2: The arrow is on the third line past the long line indicating 101 degrees. The reading is 101.6°F.

PRACTICAL PROBLEMS

Use the diagram to complete problems 1 to 10. For each temperature reading, locate the line on the diagram that represents the reading. Draw an arrow to the correct line and put the number of the problem by each arrow.

Example A: 99.8°

1.   98.2°

2.   100.6°

3.   95.0°

4.   97.8°

5.   101.4°

6.   96.2°

7.   102.6°

8.   104.4°

9.   99.2°

10.   94.8°

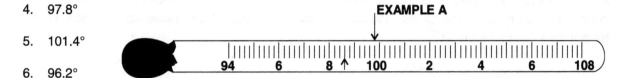

Use the diagram to complete problems 11 to 20. Write the correct temperature shown by the arrows for each problem.

Example B: The reading shown is 94.4°.

11.   _____

12.   _____

13.   _____

14.   _____

15.   _____

16.   _____

17. _____

18. _____

19. _____

20. _____

Unit 31 SPHYGMOMANOMETER GAUGES

BASIC PRINCIPLES OF READING SPHYGMOMANOMETER GAUGES

A sphygmomanometer is an instrument calibrated for measuring blood pressure (BP) in millimeters (mm) of mercury (Hg). There are two main types of sphygmomanometer gauges, mercury and aneroid.

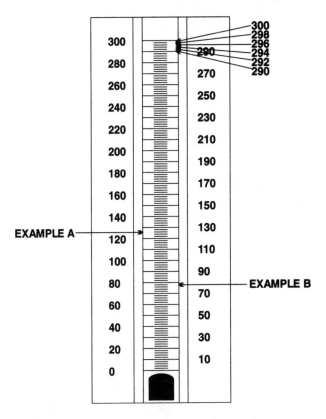

The mercury sphygmomanometer has a long column of mercury. Each line on the gauge represents two millimeters of mercury (mm Hg). If it is calibrated correctly, the level of mercury should be at zero when viewed at eye level. Since blood pressure is recorded as the pressure drops in the gauge, it is best to learn to read the gauge in a backward direction. Note the example starting with 300 mm Hg and ending with 290 mm Hg.

Example A: Since the arrow is two lines below the 130 reading, read as 130 − 2 − 2 = 126. The reading is 126 mm Hg.

Example B: This is one line below 80, so the reading is 80 − 2 = 78 mm Hg.

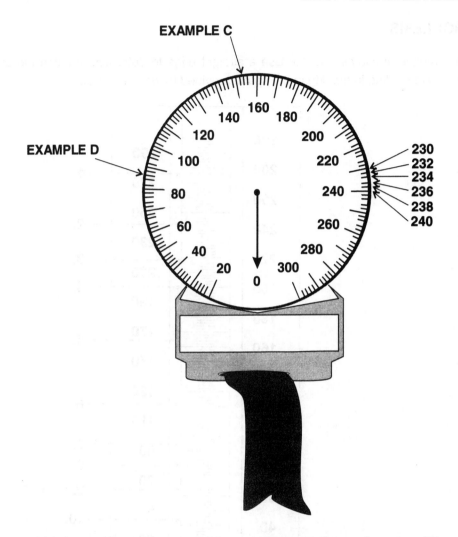

The aneroid sphygmomanometer gauge does not have a column of mercury. It is calibrated equivalent to mm Hg, and each line represents 2 mm Hg. It is important to note that long lines represent a multiple of ten. Odd multiples of ten, such as 30 and 50, are not written on the scale. Since readings are recorded as the pressure drops, it is best to learn to read the gauge in a backward direction.

Example C: This reading is 4 lines below the 160 mark, so it equals 160 − 2 − 2 − 2 − 2 = 152 mm Hg.

Example D: This reading is 2 lines below the 90 mark, so it equals 90 − 2 − 2 = 86 mm Hg.

PRACTICAL PROBLEMS

Use the diagram to complete problems 1 to 10. Use a straight edge to determine the line the arrow indicates. Place the correct reading in mm Hg in the space provided by each number.

1. _____

2. _____

3. _____

4. _____

5. _____

6. _____

7. _____

8. _____

9. _____

10. _____

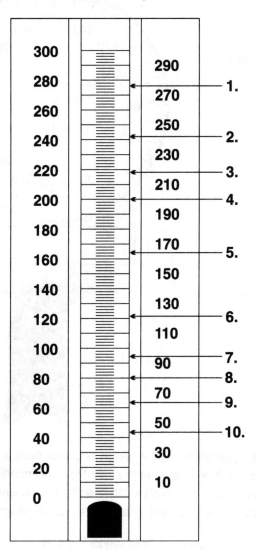

Use the diagram to complete problems 11 to 20. Use a straight edge to determine the line the arrow indicates. Place the correct reading in mm Hg in the space provided by each number.

11. _____

12. _____

13. _____

14. _____

15. _____

16. _____

17. _____

18. _____

19. _____

20. _____

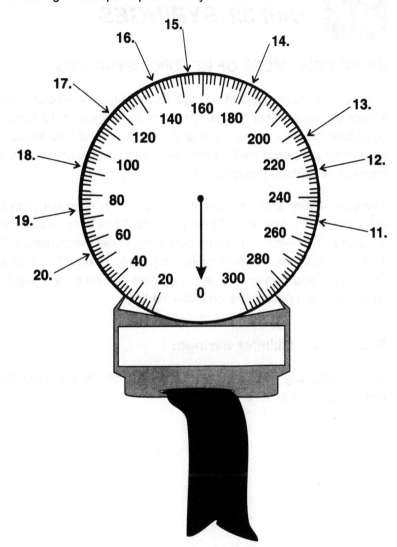

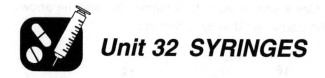

Unit 32 SYRINGES

BASIC PRINCIPLES OF READING SYRINGES

Syringes are measuring devices used for *parenteral* or injectable medications. Common injection routes include intramuscular or IM (into a muscle), intravenous or IV (into a vein), subcutaneous or SC (into the subcutaneous layer of tissue just under the skin), and intradermal or ID (just under the top layer of the skin). Most parenteral medications are in a liquid or solution form. They are packaged in dosage vials, ampules, or prefilled syringes.

There are many different types of syringes. The most common types are 3 milliliters (ml) or cubic centimeters (cc), 5 ml or cc, 10 ml or cc, and 20 ml or cc syringes. It is important to remember that 1 ml is equal to 1 cc—that a ml and a cc are the same measurement. The 3-ml syringe is used for IM and some SC injections. The 5-ml syringe is usually used for IV injections or venipunctures to obtain blood. The 10-ml and larger syringes are used for irrigations, aspirations (withdrawing fluids or air), venipunctures, IV injections, and tube feedings.

Reading a 3-Milliliter Syringe:

Before using any syringe, it is important to check the calibrations and determine what each line represents. Look at the 3-ml syringe.

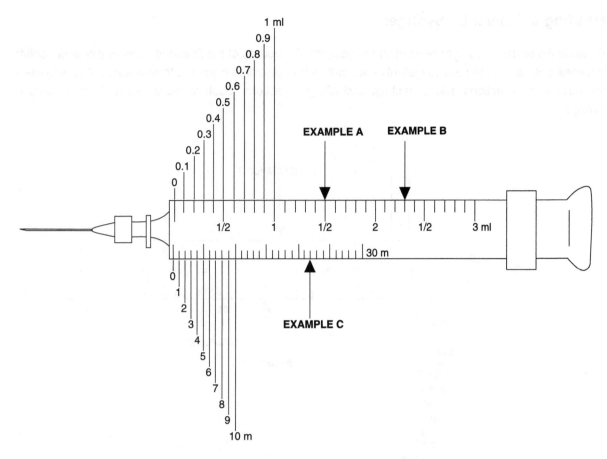

This 3-ml syringe contains calibration scales for both milliliters (ml) and the largely obsolete minim (m) scale of the apothecaries' system. The first long line at the base of the syringe where it joins with the needle represents the zero mark for both of the scales. For the ml scale, each line above the zero line represents 0.1 or ¹⁄₁₀ of a ml. Longer lines represent the 0.5-ml (or ½-ml) marks, and the 1-ml levels. The minim side of the scale is divided into 1 m intervals. Longer lines mark the 5, 10, 15, 20, 25, and 30 m levels. On most syringes the minims are not marked except for the final number, in this case 30 m. In this syringe 16 m = 1 ml. To read a syringe, start at the base end of the syringe and read up toward the plunger end.

Example A: The arrow above the syringe is pointing to the 1½-ml mark. It is read as 1½ or 1.5 ml.

Example B: The arrow above the syringe is pointing to the third line past the 2-ml mark. It is read as 2³⁄₁₀ or 2.3 ml.

Example C: The arrow below the syringe is pointing to the second line past the 20-m mark. It is read as 22 m.

Reading a Tuberculin Syringe:

A tuberculin or low-dose syringe is used to inject small amounts of medications such as pediatric (child) dosages and heparin (an anticoagulant or substance that prevents the blood from clotting). It is also used for intradermal injections, allergy testing, and allergy injections. Look at the diagram of the tuberculin syringe.

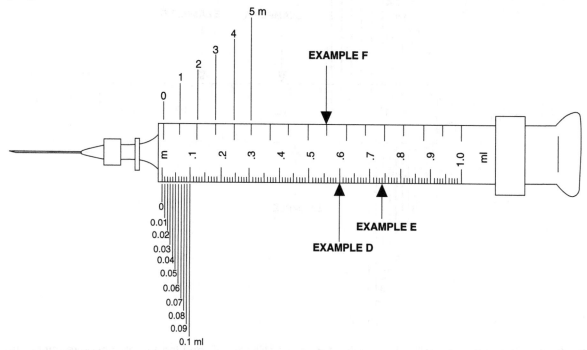

This tuberculin syringe contains calibration scales for both milliliters (ml) and the largely obsolete minim (m) scales of the apothecaries' system. The first long line at the base of the syringe where it joins with the needle represents the zero mark for both of the scales. The bottom scale is for ml and the syringe contains a total of 1 ml. Each line above the zero line represents 0.01 or $\frac{1}{100}$ of a ml. Longer lines represent the 0.1-ml (or $\frac{1}{10}$-ml) marks. The top scale is minims. Each line represents 1 m. The minims are not marked with numbers. In this syringe 16 m = 1 ml. It is important not to read the m scale if you are calculating the dosage in ml. Always make sure you are reading the correct scale or a serious medication error could occur. To read the syringe, start at the base end and read up toward the plunger end.

Example D: The arrow below the syringe is pointing to the 0.6-ml mark. It is read as $\frac{6}{10}$ or 0.6 ml.

Example E: The arrow below the syringe is pointing to the fourth line past the 0.7-ml mark. It is read as $\frac{74}{100}$ or $\frac{37}{50}$ or 0.74 ml.

Example F: The arrow above the syringe is pointing to the ninth line past the zero mark. It is read as 9 m.

Reading an Insulin Syringe:

Patients with a condition called diabetes mellitus, or "sugar," use insulin syringes to measure the correct dose of insulin needed. Diabetes is a metabolic disorder caused by a lack of or insufficient production of insulin, a hormone produced by the pancreas. Insulin helps the body transport glucose, a form of sugar, from the bloodstream into body cells where the glucose is used to produce energy. If the person does not take insulin, the sugar builds up in the bloodstream and leads to serious complications including death.

Insulin is a medication that is used as a substitute for the missing hormone. It is available as 100 units (U) per milliliter (ml) of solution. Different sizes of insulin syringes are used, depending on the dosage of insulin the patient requires. Look at the 30-U, 50-U, and 100-U insulin syringes.

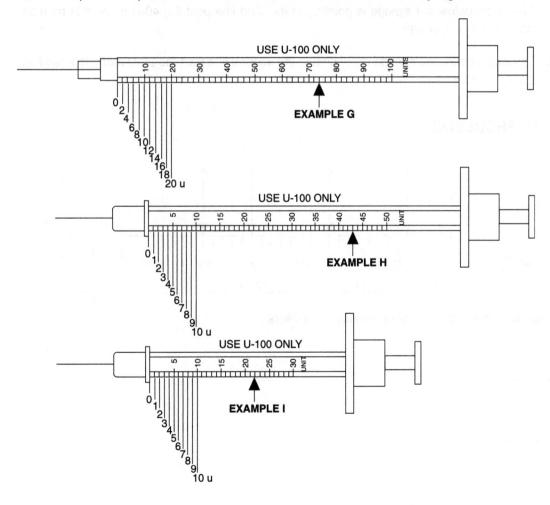

Insulin syringes are used only for measuring insulin since they are calibrated in units. Both the 30-U and 50-U syringes are calibrated in units. Each line indicates 1 U. Every 5 units is indicated by numbers such as 5, 10, 15, and so forth. These syringes are used for small doses of insulin so exact amounts can be measured accurately. The 100-U syringe is used for larger amounts of insulin. Each line indicates 2 U. Every 10 units is indicated by numbers such as 10, 20, 30, and so forth. If a patient has to take 14 U of insulin, the 30-U syringe would be used. If a person needs 37 U of insulin, a 50-U syringe is preferred. For dosages higher than 50 U, the 100-U syringe would be used. To read any of the syringes, start at the base end and read up toward the plunger end.

Example G: The arrow below the syringe is pointing to the second line past the 70-U mark. It is read as 70 + 2 + 2 or 74 U.

Example H: The arrow below the syringe is pointing to the third line past the 40-U mark. It is read as 40 + 1 + 1 + 1 or 43 U.

Example I: The arrow below the syringe is pointing to the second line past the 20-U mark. It is read as 20 + 1 + 1 or 22 U.

PRACTICAL PROBLEMS

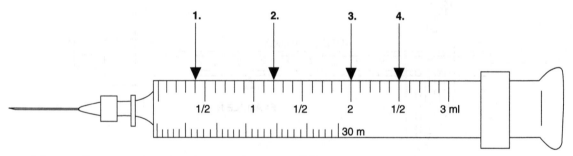

Record the readings noted on the above syringe in milliliters.

1. _____

2. _____

3. _____

4. _____

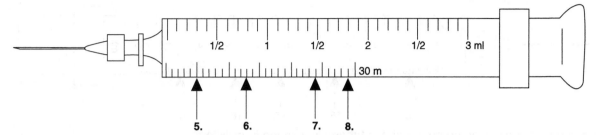

Record the readings noted on the above syringe in minims.

5. _____

6. _____

7. _____

8. _____

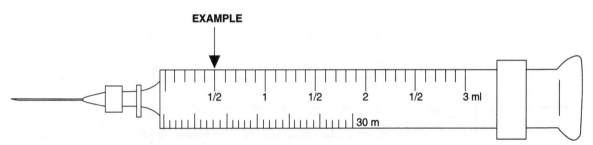

On the above syringe, draw an arrow to the correct area on the syringe for the measurements shown. Put the number of the problem by the arrow.

Example: The arrow is drawn to the 0.5-ml (or ½-ml) mark on the syringe.

9. 1 ml

10. 1.7 or 1⁷⁄₁₀ ml

11. 2.1 or 2¹⁄₁₀ ml

12. 8 m

13. 11 m

14. 18 m

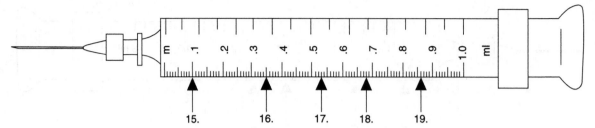

Record the readings noted on the above tuberculin syringe in milliliters.

15. _____

16. _____

17. _____

18. _____

19. _____

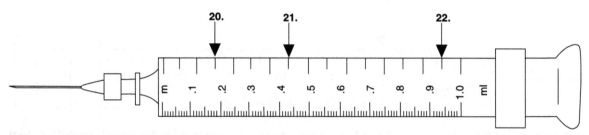

Record the readings noted on the above tuberculin syringe in minims.

20. _____

21. _____

22. _____

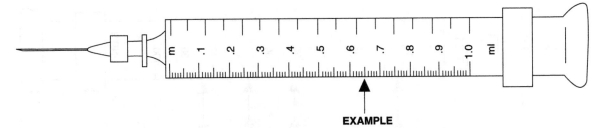

EXAMPLE

On the above syringe, draw an arrow to the correct area on the syringe for the measurements shown. Put the number of the problem by the arrow.

Example: The arrow is drawn to the 0.65-ml (or $^{13}/_{20}$-ml) mark on the syringe.

23. 0.04 ml

24. 0.59 ml

25. 0.94 ml

26. 0.37 ml

27. $^{1}/_{4}$ ml

28. $^{41}/_{50}$ ml

29. 11 m

30. 1 m

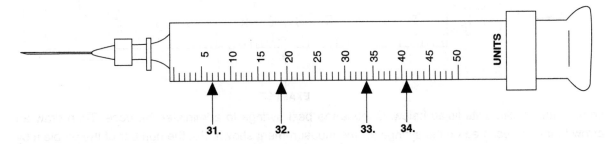

31.   32.   33. 34.

Record the readings noted on the 50-U insulin syringe.

31. _____

32. _____

33. _____

34. _____

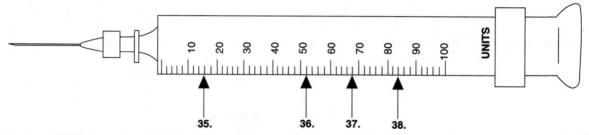

35.   36.   37.   38.

Record the readings noted on the 100-U insulin syringe.

35.   _____

36.   _____

37.   _____

38.   _____

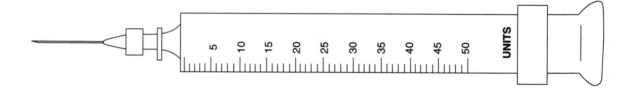

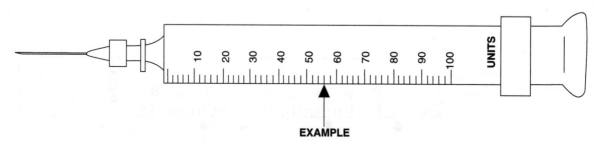

EXAMPLE

Look at the insulin units listed below. Choose the best syringe to administer the dose. Then draw an arrow to the correct area on the syringe for the measurement shown. Put the number of the problem by the arrow.

Example: An order for 56 U of insulin would require a 100-U syringe. The arrow is drawn to the 56-U mark on the 100-U syringe.

39.   11 U

40.   94 U

41.   47 U

42.   38 U

43.   66 U

44.   72 U

45.   29 U

46.   88 U

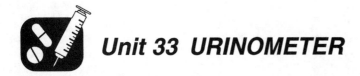

Unit 33 URINOMETER

BASIC PRINCIPLES OF READING A URINOMETER

Specific gravity (SpGr) of urine is a measurement of the weight of urine compared with the weight of an equal amount of distilled water. The normal range for specific gravity is 1.010 to 1.025. A urinometer is one instrument used to measure specific gravity of urine. The urinometer is a float with a calibrated stem that is placed in urine with a spinning motion.

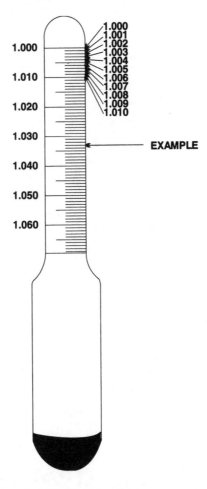

Each calibration on the urinometer float is in thousandths. The top line represents 1.000, and each small line below it represents 0.001. Note the readings shown on the diagram.

Example: Since the arrow in the example is pointing to the third line below 1.030, the reading would be 1.030 + 0.001 + 0.001 + 0.001 = 1.033.

PRACTICAL PROBLEMS

Use the diagram to complete problems 1 to 16. Use a straight edge to determine what line on the urinometer float each arrow indicates. Write the correct reading in the space provided by each number.

1. _____

2. _____

3. _____

4. _____

5. _____

6. _____

7. _____

8. _____

9. _____

10. _____

11. _____

12. _____

13. _____

14. _____

15. _____

16. _____

17. _____

18. _____

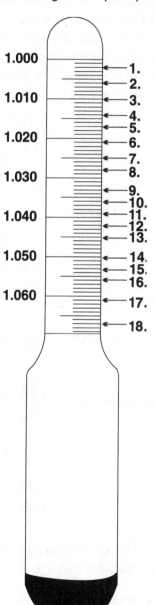

Unit 34 MICROHEMATOCRIT CENTRIFUGE

BASIC PRINCIPLES OF READING A MICROHEMATOCRIT CENTRIFUGE

A hematocrit (hct) is a blood test that measures the volume or percent of erythrocytes (red blood cells or RBC) in the blood. A microhematocrit centrifuge is an instrument that is used to calculate hematocrit. It spins a tube or tubes of blood at 10,000 revolutions per minute with a centrifugal (driving away from the center) force. This force separates the blood into three main layers: red blood cells, white blood cells, and plasma. The layer of red blood cells is on the bottom of the tube. By using the graphic reading device on the microhematocrit centrifuge, the percentage of red blood cells can be measured.

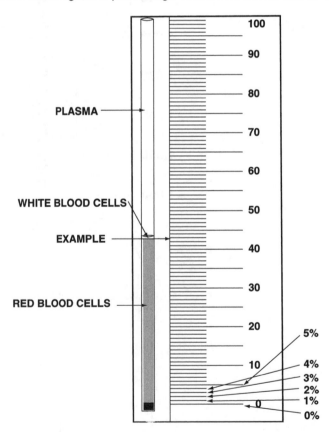

The scale on the microhematocrit centrifuge is in percent (%). The numbers represent 0% to 100%. Each line represents 1 percent. Note the readings shown on the diagram.

Example: Since the example arrow is 3 lines above the 40% mark, the reading would be 40 + 1 + 1 + 1 = 43%. The reading should always contain the percent sign.

PRACTICAL PROBLEMS

Use the diagram to complete problems 1 to 20. Use a straight edge to determine what line on the microhematocrit centrifuge each arrow indicates. Write the correct reading in the space provided by each number.

1. _____
2. _____
3. _____
4. _____
5. _____
6. _____
7. _____
8. _____
9. _____
10. _____
11. _____
12. _____
13. _____
14. _____
15. _____
16. _____
17. _____
18. _____
19. _____
20. _____

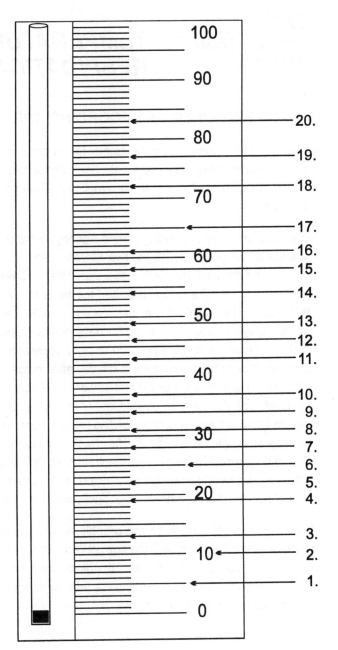

Graphs and Charts

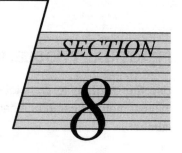

Unit 35 TEMPERATURE, PULSE, AND RESPIRATION (TPR) GRAPHICS

BASIC PRINCIPLES OF RECORDING TPR GRAPHICS

Graphics are special records used for recording temperature, pulse, and respiration (TPR) measurements. They are used most often in hospitals and long-term care facilities, but can be used in medical offices and other health care facilities. They present a visual diagram of variations in a patient's vital signs.

Graphic charts vary depending on the agency, but they all contain the same basic information. Review the sample graphic shown. At the top, there are spaces to fill in the patient's name, doctor, room number, and other information. Below this, there are blocks to represent days of the week. Most graphics contain 7- or 8-day blocks. A space is provided for the date. On a hospital graphic, a line is provided for days in the hospital. The day of admission is noted as "ADM," and the next day is day 1 or the first full day in the hospital. Days "P.O. or P.P." stand for days postoperative (after surgery) or postpartum (after delivery of a baby). The day of surgery is noted as "OR" (operating room) or "Surg" (surgery) followed by a 1 in the next day block to represent the first full day after surgery. The day of delivery of a baby is shown as "Del" with the next day as day 1 or the first day after delivery. Numbers continue in sequence for each following day. Each day block is then divided into time segments, usually four-hour intervals. Along the side of the graphic, there are sections for recording temperature, pulse, and respiration (TPR). For temperature, the readings start with 96 and go to 106. Each line represents 0.5 degrees, and would read 96, 96.5, 97, 97.5, and so forth. For pulse and respiration each line represents 5. Lines represent 10, 15, 20, and so forth, but only the even numbers are listed on the chart. At the bottom of the graphic, there are areas for recording blood pressure (BP), weight (wt), intake and output (I & O) totals, and other similar information.

When notations are made on the graphic, it is important to find the right day and time column. Move down the correct column until the correct reading for either temperature, pulse, or respiration is located. A dot is then placed in the middle of the block between the time lines. Note the position of the dots in the example shown. To connect readings, a ruler or straight edge should be used. This is a legal record and must be accurate, neat, and legible.

GRAPHIC CHART

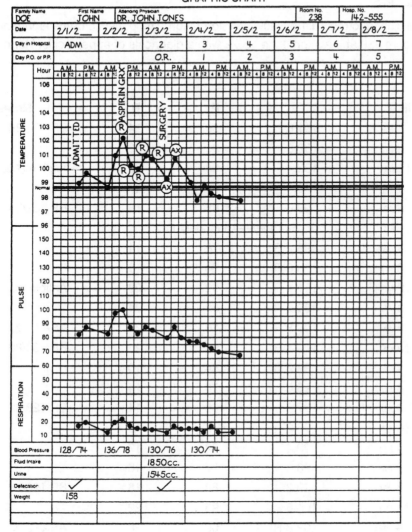

(Courtesy of Physician's Record Company, Berwyn, IL)

For pulse and respiration, only dots are used to record a measurement. A plain dot in the temperature column indicates an oral temperature measurement. If a rectal measurement is recorded, an ⓡ is placed by the dot. If an axillary measurement is recorded, an ⒶⓍ is placed by the dot.

In some agencies, drugs that alter or change the temperature or other vital signs are noted on the graphic. A common example is aspirin (ASA) that acts to lower temperature. The name of the drug is written in the correct time column as shown on the sample graphic. Other events may also be recorded on the graphic in the same manner. Examples include surgery, isolation, admission, and discharge.

PRACTICAL PROBLEMS

1. Use the blank graphic chart to record the following information. The patient's name is Virginia Clay. She is admitted to room 238 at 4 P.M. on June 15, –, with a diagnosis of appendicitis. Her doctor is Dr. Pease.

Date	Time	T	P	R	Notes
6/15/–	4 PM	101.8	96	24	BP 134/88
	8 PM	102.6	98	26	
	12 MN	103.4	108	28	Aspirin (ASA) Gr V
6/16/–	4 AM	100.4	94	22	
	8 AM	99.6	88	16	BP 132/84
	12 Noon	Surgery—Appendectomy			
	4 PM	98.2 R	78	14	
	8 PM	98.6 R	84	16	
	12 MN	101.4 R	92	20	Antibiotics
6/17/–	4 AM	102.6 R	98	24	
	8 AM	103.8 R	110	24	ASA Gr X
	12 Noon	100.4 R	94	20	BP 130/86
	4 PM	99.2 R	84	16	
	8 PM	98.8	76	14	
6/18/–	8 AM	97.6	68	14	BP 128/82
	12 Noon	98.2	75	15	
	4 PM	99.4	82	17	
	8 PM	98.8	77	16	
6/19/–	8 AM	99.2	88	18	BP 126/78
	12 Noon	101.6	98	22	
	4 PM	102.8 R	106	26	ASA Gr X
	8 PM	100.6 R	94	20	
	12 MN	99.2 R	86	17	
6/20/–	8 AM	98.8	74	14	BP 124/76
	12 Noon	98.8	81	15	
	4 PM	99.4	85	17	
	8 PM	98.6	82	16	
6/21/–	8 AM	97.8	74	14	BP 122/78
	12 Noon	98.4	81	16	Discharged

GRAPHIC CHART

Family Name		First Name		Attending Physician			Room No.		Hosp. No.	

Date								
Day in Hospital								
Day P O or P P								

	Hour	AM / PM	AM / PM	AM / PM	AM / PM	AM / PM	AM / PM	AM / PM	AM / PM
		4 8 12 4 8 12	4 8 12 4 8 12	4 8 12 4 8 12	4 8 12 4 8 12	4 8 12 4 8 12	4 8 12 4 8 12	4 8 12 4 8 12	4 8 12 4 8 12

TEMPERATURE

106
105
104
103
102
101
100
99 Normal
98
97
96

PULSE

150
140
130
120
110
100
90
80
70
60

RESPIRATION

50
40
30
20
10

Blood Pressure								
Fluid Intake								
Urine								
Defecation								
Weight								

form D-703

GRAPHIC CHART

(Courtesy of Physician's Record Company)

2.   Use the blank chart to record the following information. The patient's name is Roger Daugherty. He
is admitted to room 238 at 4 P.M. on November 28, –, with a diagnosis of mononucleosis. His doctor
is Dr. Yoder and his hospital number is 555-44.

Date	Time	T	P	R	Notes
11/28/–	4 PM	103.6 R	108	30	BP 128/80
	8 PM	104.2 R	100	26	
	12 MN	103.2 R	118	28	Aspirin Gr X
11/29/–	4 AM	101.6 R	100	24	
	8 AM	100.4 R	86	20	BP 124/84
	12 Noon	103.6 R	122	28	Aspirin Gr X
	4 PM	100.2 R	106	22	
	8 PM	104.8 R	110	32	
	12 MN	105.8 R	148	38	
11/30/–	4 AM	99.4 R	88	20	
	8 AM	98.6 R	86	18	BP 118/76
	12 Noon	98.8	80	20	
	4 PM	99.8	94	18	
	8 PM	98.2	84	16	
12/1/–	8 AM	97.6	60	12	BP 130/78
	12 Noon	98.2	66	14	
	4 PM	99.2	82	20	
	8 PM	101	98	28	
	12 MN	99.8	88	22	
12/2/–	8 AM	97.2	64	12	BP 126/76
	4 PM	98.4	86	14	
12/3/–	8 AM	100	96	24	BP 114/76
	12 Noon	99.2	86	18	
	4 PM	99.8	88	22	
	8 PM	98.8	80	18	
12/4/–	8 AM	97.8	88	16	BP 118/78
	4 PM	98.6	80	18	
12/5/–	8 AM	97.2	68	14	BP 118/76
	4 PM	98.4	80	18	Discharged

GRAPHIC CHART

| Family Name | | First Name | | Attending Physician | | | | Room No. | | Hosp. No. | |

Date	
Day in Hospital	
Day P O or P P	

	Hour	A M	P M	A M	P M	A M	P M	A M	P M	A M	P M	A M	P M	A M	P M	A M	P M
		4 8 12	4 8 12	4 8 12	4 8 12	4 8 12	4 8 12	4 8 12	4 8 12	4 8 12	4 8 12	4 8 12	4 8 12	4 8 12	4 8 12	4 8 12	4 8 12

TEMPERATURE
- 106
- 105
- 104
- 103
- 102
- 101
- 100
- 99 Normal
- 98
- 97
- 96

PULSE
- 150
- 140
- 130
- 120
- 110
- 100
- 90
- 80
- 70
- 60

RESPIRATION
- 50
- 40
- 30
- 20
- 10

Blood Pressure	
Fluid Intake	
Urine	
Defecation	
Weight	

form D-703   GRAPHIC CHART

(Courtesy of Physician's Record Company)

3. Use the blank graphic chart to record the following information. The patient's name is Jim Johnson. He is admitted to Ram Hospital, room number 238, on January 1, –. The diagnosis is hepatitis and exhaustion. Dr. Imhoff has placed the patient in isolation. His hospital number is 54-56-54. His weight when admitted is 206 pounds.

Date	Time	T	P	R	Notes
1/1/–	12 Noon	103.4 R	136	38	BP 138/84
	4 PM	104.6 R	136	46	
	8 PM	102.4 R	120	30	
	12 MN	103.2 R	130	36	Aspirin Gr XX
1/2/–	4 AM	100.4 R	116	24	
	8 AM	99.6 R	98	18	BP 124/78
	12 Noon	98.4	76	18	
	4 PM	99.6	94	24	
	8 PM	101.2	108	34	
	12 MN	103.8 R	120	42	Aspirin Gr X
1/3/–	4 AM	100.4 R	96	24	
	8 AM	99.6 R	84	18	BP 128/76
	12 Noon	99.8	88	22	
	4 PM	98.4	80	16	
	8 PM	98.8	86	18	
1/4/–	8 AM	97.2 Ax	68	12	BP 118/78
	12 Noon	98.4	76	18	
	4 PM	98.6	122	28	
	8 PM	99.4	86	18	
1/5/–	8 AM	97.6 Ax	62	14	BP 120/80
	4 PM	99.8	88	20	
	8 PM	102.6 R	94	28	Aspirin Gr XX
	12 MN	99.4 R	86	20	
1/6/–	8 AM	98.2	74	16	BP 124/72
	12 Noon	98.8	86	18	
	4 PM	98.8	90	18	
1/7/–	8 AM	97.4	64	12	BP 128/74
	8 PM	98.6	62	18	
1/8/–	8 AM	97.6	66	14	BP 120/68
	4 PM	98.4	82	12	

GRAPHIC CHART

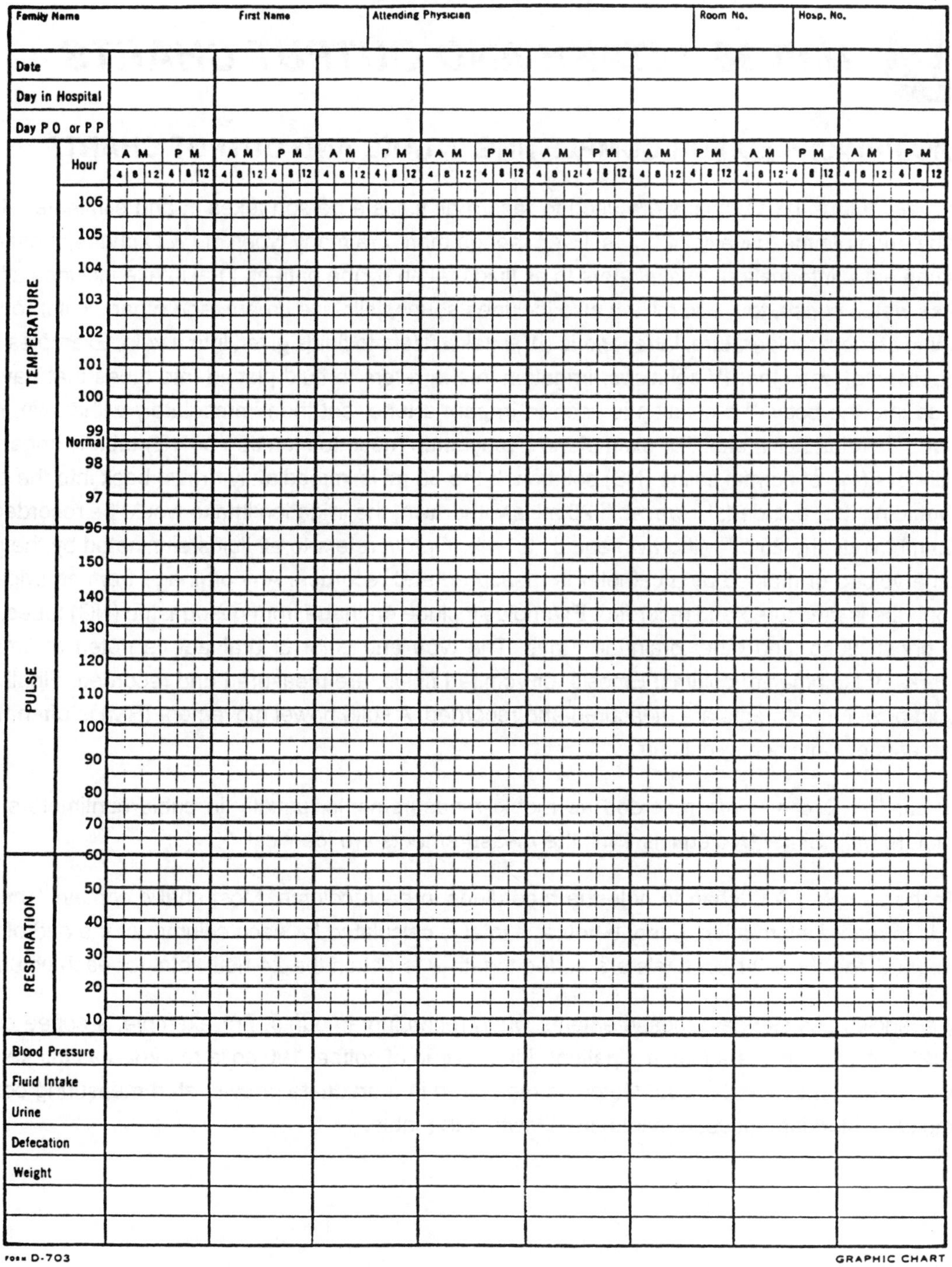

| Family Name | | | First Name | | Attending Physician | | | Room No. | | Hosp. No. | |

Date									
Day in Hospital									
Day P O or P P									

	Hour	A M	P M	A M	P M	A M	P M	A M	P M	A M	P M	A M	P M	A M	P M	A M	P M
		4 8 12	4 8 12	4 8 12	4 8 12	4 8 12	4 8 12	4 8 12	4 8 12	4 8 12	4 8 12	4 8 12	4 8 12	4 8 12	4 8 12	4 8 12	4 8 12

TEMPERATURE
106
105
104
103
102
101
100
99 Normal
98
97
96

PULSE
150
140
130
120
110
100
90
80
70
60

RESPIRATION
50
40
30
20
10

Blood Pressure									
Fluid Intake									
Urine									
Defecation									
Weight									

Form D-703

GRAPHIC CHART

(Courtesy of Physician's Record Company)

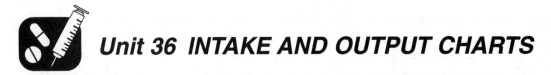

Unit 36 INTAKE AND OUTPUT CHARTS

BASIC PRINCIPLES FOR COMPLETING INTAKE AND OUTPUT CHARTS

Intake and output (I & O) charts are used to record all fluids a person takes in and eliminates during a certain period of time, usually 24 hours. Even though there are many types of I & O charts, most contain the same basic information. *Intake* refers to all fluids taken by the patient. Oral intake includes all liquids such as water, coffee, tea, and milk. It also includes soups, jello, ice cream, and other similar foods that are liquid at room temperature. Intravenous (IV) intake refers to fluids given into a vein. Examples include blood, plasma, and other IV solutions. Irrigation intake refers to fluid placed into tubes that have been inserted into the body. If a solution is used to irrigate a tube, but then immediately withdrawn, it is not recorded as irrigation intake. For example, a nasogastric (nose to stomach or NG) tube is irrigated with 50 milliliters (ml) of normal saline (NS) solution. If the 50 ml is immediately drawn back into the syringe, this would not be recorded. However, if 20 ml is withdrawn, the irrigation intake would be recorded as 30 ml (50 ml minus the 20 ml withdrawn equals 30 ml). *Output* refers to all fluids eliminated by the patient. All urine voided or drained by a catheter is measured and recorded. Any drainage from an irrigation or suction tube is measured and recorded. Examples include drainage from nasogastric (NG) tubes, hemovacs, chest tubes, and other drainage tubes. The type and color of drainage is noted at times in a "Remarks or Comments" column. Emesis, or vomited fluids, are measured and recorded. Finally, feces or liquid bowel movements are measured and recorded. A solid bowel movement (BM) is often noted in a "Remarks or Comments" column.

Fluids for I & O charts are recorded as metric measurements, usually in cubic centimeters (cc) or millimeters (ml). Since 1 cc equals 1 ml, the measurements are identical.

Study the sample I & O chart to note the recordings in each column. Most charts contain 1-hour time periods to record information. Every 8 hours, a total is calculated for each column. At the end of the 24-hour period, the three 8-hour totals are added together to obtain the 24-hour total for each column.

Most agencies use standard measurements when recording amounts. For example, a coffee cup may hold 120 cubic centimeters (cc). If a patient drinks a cup of coffee, 120 cc is recorded as intake without measuring the amount in the cup. Output is measured in a graduate or calibrated measuring container. Examples of standard measurements are shown in the table.

UNIT & MEASUREMENT	CONTAINER & MEASUREMENT
15 drops (gtt) = 1 cc or ml	1 juice glass = 120 cc or ml
1 teaspoon (tsp) = 5 cc or ml	1 water glass = 180 cc or ml
1 tablespoon (tbsp) = 15 cc or ml	1 large glass = 240 cc or ml
1 ounce (oz) = 30 cc or ml	1 coffee cup = 120 cc or ml
1 pint (pt) = 500 cc or ml	1 small bowl = 120 cc or ml
1 quart (qt) = 1000 cc or ml	1 soup bowl = 200 cc or ml

INTAKE AND OUTPUT RECORD													

Family Name			First Name	Attending Physician		Room No.	Hosp. No.
JOHNSON, ROBERT				DR. MIKE SMITH		238	54-3201

Date 9/30	INTAKE				OUTPUT				OTHER				REMARKS
TIME	Oral	I.V.	Blood		Urine	Tube	Emesis	Feces					
7 - 8 a.m.	100												
8 - 9 a.m.	320						200						EMESIS– GREEN LIQUID
9 - 10 a.m.					420								
10 - 11 a.m.	100												
11 - 12 noon				10									NG IRRIGATION: NS
12 - 1 p.m.	240				310								
1 - 2 p.m.		850				200							NASOGASTRIC GOLD – BROWN
2 - 3 p.m.	60												
8 HOUR TOTAL	820	850		10	730	200	200						
3 - 4 p.m.													
4 - 5 p.m.	320	150					120						BROWN LIQUID
5 - 6 p.m.					280								
6 - 7 p.m.	180												
7 - 8 p.m.													
8 - 9 p.m.	100												
9 - 10 p.m.		500				240							NASOGASTRIC BROWNISH
10 - 11 p.m.					310								
8 HOUR TOTAL	600	650			590	240		120					
11 - 12 p.m.													
12 - 1 a.m.				10									NG IRRIGATION: NS
1 - 2 a.m.	180				420								
2 - 3 a.m.													
3 - 4 a.m.							650						EMESIS– GREEN LIQUID
4 - 5 a.m.													
5 - 6 a.m.		600				180							NASOGASTRIC GOLD – BROWN
6 - 7 a.m.	100				380								
8 HOUR TOTAL	280	600		10	800	180	650						
24 HOUR TOTAL	1700	2100		20	2120	620	850	120					
	TOTAL INTAKE 3820				TOTAL OUTPUT 3710								

(Courtesy of Physician's Record Company)

PRACTICAL PROBLEMS

1. Study the sample chart to note how measurements should be recorded. At the end of each 8-hour period, add the 8-hour totals for each column. When all information is recorded, add the three 8-hour totals together to obtain the 24-hour total for each column. Then add all of the 24-hour intake columns together to obtain the "Total Intake" and all of the 24-hour output columns together to obtain the "Total Output."

    Use the blank I & O chart to record the following information. The patient, Dennis Bartlett, is in room 238 after abdominal surgery. A nasogastric (NG) tube is in place and connected to a low suction drainage unit. An intravenous (IV) solution is infusing into a vein.

7 AM	Drank 1 large glass of water Voided 230 cc of urine
8 AM	Ate breakfast: 1 juice glass of tomato juice, 2 cups of coffee, and 1 soup bowl of oatmeal (*Hint:* Add totals together and record as one entry.)
9 AM	Nasogastric (NG) tube irrigated with 30 cc normal saline (NS) and 20 cc withdrawn to syringe
10 AM	Voided 180 cc of urine Drank 1 large glass of ginger ale
12 Noon	Ate lunch: 1 juice glass of apple juice, ½ soup bowl of broth, 1 small bowl of jello, ½ small bowl of ice cream, and 1½ cups of tea
1 PM	Vomited 260 cc of light brown emesis
2 PM	Absorbed 540 cc of IV solution Nasogastric (NG) drainage jar emptied and measured: 110 cc of light yellow clear liquid Voided 220 cc of urine
4 PM	Drank ½ large glass of ginger ale Expelled 160 cc of light brown liquid stool (feces)
6 PM	Ate dinner: ¾ soup bowl of broth, ½ juice glass of apple juice, ½ small bowl jello, ¾ large glass of milk, ½ cup coffee
7 PM	Voided 270 cc of urine
8 PM	Vomited 180 cc of light yellow emesis NG tube irrigated with 30 cc of NS solution with no return of solution
9 PM	Drank 3 tablespoons of ginger ale Absorbed 1 pint of blood in IV
10 PM	Drank 2 tablespoons of ginger ale Absorbed 150 cc of NS in IV NG drainage jar emptied and measured: 220 cc of light golden-brown clear liquid
11 PM	Drank 4 tablespoons of ginger ale Voided 280 cc of urine
1 AM	Drank 1 juice glass of ginger ale
4 AM	Drank 1 large glass of water Voided 180 cc of urine NG tube irrigated with 30 cc of NS solution and 10 cc returned to syringe

6 AM   Absorbed 450 cc of NS IV solution
         Drank ¾ large glass of water
         NG drainage jar emptied and measured: 140 cc of light yellow clear liquid

INTAKE AND OUTPUT RECORD													
Family Name			First Name		Attending Physician			Room No.		Hosp. No.			
Date	INTAKE				OUTPUT				OTHER				REMARKS
TIME	Oral	I.V.	Blood		Urine	Tube	Emesis	Feces					
7 - 8 a.m.													
8 - 9 a.m.													
9 - 10 a.m.													
10 - 11 a.m.													
11 - 12 noon													
12 - 1 p.m.													
1 - 2 p.m.													
2 - 3 p.m.													
8 HOUR TOTAL													
3 - 4 p.m.													
4 - 5 p.m.													
5 - 6 p.m.													
6 - 7 p.m.													
7 - 8 p.m.													
8 - 9 p.m.													
9 - 10 p.m.													
10 - 11 p.m.													
8 HOUR TOTAL													
11 - 12 p.m.													
12 - 1 a.m.													
1 - 2 a.m.													
2 - 3 a.m.													
3 - 4 a.m.													
4 - 5 a.m.													
5 - 6 a.m.													
6 - 7 a.m.													
8 HOUR TOTAL													
24 HOUR TOTAL	TOTAL INTAKE				TOTAL OUTPUT								

(Courtesy of Physician's Record Company)

2. Use the blank I & O chart to record the following information. Make sure you total all 8-hour and 24-hour columns when the information has been recorded. Totals must also be obtained for "Total Intake" and "Total Output."

Tamika Perry, a patient of Dr. Kowalski, had a gastrectomy (surgical removal of the stomach). A nasogastric (NG) tube is in place to drain all fluids. It is connected to suction and irrigated at times. An intravenous (IV) solution is providing liquid intake. Oral intake is limited to sips of ginger ale or water and ice cubes.

a. NG tube was irrigated with normal saline (NS) as follows:

7 AM	10 cc	9 PM	25 cc with 10 cc withdrawn
11 AM	10 cc	1 AM	10 cc
4 PM	10 cc	4 AM	20 cc with 5 cc withdrawn

b. IV was absorbed as follows:

12 Noon	400 cc	10 PM	200 cc
2 PM	150 cc	3 AM	400 cc
8 PM	500 cc	6 AM	200 cc

c. Urine output was as follows:

9 AM	400 cc	9 PM	550 cc
1 PM	250 cc	1 AM	400 cc
5 PM	375 cc	5 AM	200 cc

d. The patient had greenish liquid stool as follows:

11 AM	300 cc	5 PM	200 cc	3 AM	750 cc

e. The NG tube suction jar was emptied on each shift. Measurements were as follows:

2 PM	780 cc greenish liquid
10 PM	550 cc golden-brown liquid
6 AM	625 cc golden-brown liquid

f. Water intake was as follows:

8 AM	2 tbsp	12 Midnight	2 tbsp
1 PM	1 tbsp	3 AM	1 tbsp
5 PM	3 tbsp		

g. Sips of ginger ale were taken as follows:

9 AM	½ juice glass	8 PM	1 oz
12 Noon	½ large glass	1 AM	2 oz
6 PM	1 juice glass	4 AM	½ water glass

h. The patient vomited several times. Amounts were as follows:

2 PM	100 cc clear liquid
9 PM	130 cc reddish-brown liquid
5 PM	200 cc golden-green liquid

i. Ice cubes were given as follows: (*Note:* 1 ice cube = 5 cc.)

2 ice cubes at 7 AM, 12 Noon, 4 PM, 10 PM, and 2 AM

INTAKE AND OUTPUT RECORD														
Family Name		First Name		Attending Physician			Room No.			Hosp. No.				
Date	**INTAKE**				**OUTPUT**					**OTHER**				**REMARKS**
TIME	Oral	I.V.	Blood		Urine	Tube	Emesis	Feces						
7 - 8 a.m.														
8 - 9 a.m.														
9 - 10 a.m.														
10 - 11 a.m.														
11 - 12 noon														
12 - 1 p.m.														
1 - 2 p.m.														
2 - 3 p.m.														
8 HOUR TOTAL														
3 - 4 p.m.														
4 - 5 p.m.														
5 - 6 p.m.														
6 - 7 p.m.														
7 - 8 p.m.														
8 - 9 p.m.														
9 - 10 p.m.														
10 - 11 p.m.														
8 HOUR TOTAL														
11 - 12 p.m.														
12 - 1 a.m.														
1 - 2 a.m.														
2 - 3 a.m.														
3 - 4 a.m.														
4 - 5 a.m.														
5 - 6 a.m.														
6 - 7 a.m.														
8 HOUR TOTAL														
24 HOUR TOTAL														
	TOTAL INTAKE				TOTAL OUTPUT									

(Courtesy of Physician's Record Company)

3. Use the blank I & O chart to record the following information. Make sure you total all 8-hour and 24-hour columns when the information has been recorded. Totals must also be obtained for "Total Intake" and "Total Output."

Maranda O'Connor, a patient of Dr. Schmidt, was admitted to intensive care at Ram Hospital with a high fever and nausea and vomiting. A nasogastric (NG) tube was inserted and connected to suction drainage. An intravenous (IV) infusion was started. She was allowed clear liquids and ice chips by mouth.

a. IV of 5% D/W (Dextrose in Water) was absorbed as follows:

10 AM	200 cc	8 PM	450 cc	2 AM	100 cc
2 PM	550 cc	10 PM	100 cc	6 AM	200 cc

b. The NG tube as irrigated with NS (normal saline) as follows:

10 AM	25 cc with 15 cc withdrawn	9 PM	35 cc with 25 cc withdrawn
1 PM	30 cc with 20 cc withdrawn	2 AM	15 cc with 5 cc withdrawn
5 PM	15 cc	5 AM	25 cc with 15 cc withdrawn

c. NG tube drainage was measured as follows:

    2 PM 550 cc greenish-brown
   10 PM 200 cc golden-brown
    6 AM 450 cc greenish

d. Meals were as follows:

     8 AM   Breakfast: 1 glass juice, ½ small bowl broth, 1 small bowl jello
    12 Noon Lunch: 1 large glass juice, 1 soup bowl broth, 2 small bowls jello
     5 PM   Supper: 1 glass juice, 1 soup bowl broth, 1 small bowl jello

e. Ice cubes were given as follows: (*Note:* 1 ice cube = 5 cc.)

    1 ice cube at 9 AM, 11 AM, 3 PM, and 10 PM
    2 ice cubes at 12 Noon, 4 PM, 12 Midnight, and 2 AM
    3 ice cubes at 2 PM and 5 PM

f. Ginger ale was given as follows:

    1 juice glass at 10 AM and 7 PM
    ½ water glass at 1 PM and 9 PM

g. Water was given as follows:

    ½ water glass at 7 AM and 6 PM
    1 water glass at 1 AM and 5 AM

h. Urine output was as follows:

10 AM	400 cc	10 PM	Patient incontinent, qs (quantity sufficient)
1 PM	550 cc	1 AM	500 cc
5 PM	400 cc	4 AM	650 cc

i. Emesis was expelled as follows:

    9 AM 200 cc clear liquid
    7 PM 300 cc brownish liquid

j. Stool was expelled as follows:

    8 AM 1 formed brown stool
    7 PM 200 cc brown liquid
    2 AM 300 cc brown liquid

INTAKE AND OUTPUT RECORD														
Family Name			**First Name**		**Attending Physician**			**Room No.**			**Hosp. No.**			
Date	**INTAKE**				**OUTPUT**				**OTHER**				**REMARKS**	
TIME	Oral	I.V.	Blood		Urine	Tube	Emesis	Feces						
7 - 8 a.m.														
8 - 9 a.m.														
9 - 10 a.m.														
10 - 11 a.m.														
11 - 12 noon														
12 - 1 p.m.														
1 - 2 p.m.														
2 - 3 p.m.														
8 HOUR TOTAL														
3 - 4 p.m.														
4 - 5 p.m.														
5 - 6 p.m.														
6 - 7 p.m.														
7 - 8 p.m.														
8 - 9 p.m.														
9 - 10 p.m.														
10 - 11 p.m.														
8 HOUR TOTAL														
11 - 12 p.m.														
12 - 1 a.m.														
1 - 2 a.m.														
2 - 3 a.m.														
3 - 4 a.m.														
4 - 5 a.m.														
5 - 6 a.m.														
6 - 7 a.m.														
8 HOUR TOTAL														
24 HOUR TOTAL														
	TOTAL INTAKE				**TOTAL OUTPUT**									

(Courtesy of Physician's Record Company)

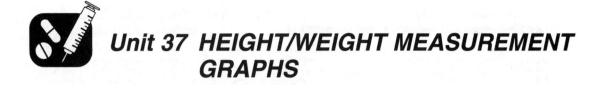

Unit 37 HEIGHT/WEIGHT MEASUREMENT GRAPHS

BASIC PRINCIPLES FOR COMPLETING HEIGHT/WEIGHT MEASUREMENT GRAPHS

Height/weight (Ht/Wt) measurement graphs are used to record and evaluate the physical growth rate of infants and children. Standard graphs are usually designed for specific sex and age groups. Different graphs are used for boys and girls since normal growth rates vary according to sex. Graphs are also available for ages birth to 36 months and ages 2 years to 18 years. Most graphs contain a section that shows normal patterns of growth and the percentile of infants or children that follow the particular growth pattern.

The sample graph shown on the next page is for a boy from birth to 36 months. The age in months is recorded at the top of the graph with each vertical line representing one month. Length is recorded on the top section of the graph. It can be recorded for both inches (in) and centimeters (cm). The scale for inches is on the outer left column. Each line represents ¼ in and would read 15, 15¼, 15²⁄₄ or 15½, 15¾, 16, 16¼, and 16½ in. Next to the inch scale is the centimeter (cm) scale. Each line represents 1 cm and would read 40, 41, 42, 43, 44, and 45 cm. Weight is recorded on the bottom section of the graph. It can be recorded for both pounds (lb) and kilograms (kg). The scale for pounds is on the outer left column at the bottom of the chart, and the outer right column at the top of the chart. Each line on the pound scale represents ½ lb and would read 4, 4½, 5, 5½, and 6 lb. The scale for kilograms is on the inner left column at the bottom of the chart, and the inner right column at the top of the chart. Each line on the kilogram scale represents 0.2 kg and would read 2, 2.2, 2.4, 2.6, 2.8, and 3 kg.

After an infant's measurements are recorded on the graph, it is easy to determine that the infant is progressing well in a normal growth pattern. The infant shown is close to the 50th percentile line, which means that he is larger than 50% of infants his age, but smaller than 50% of infants his age. A graphic chart is a legal record. All entries must be accurate, neat, and legible. Most graphic charts are completed in blue or black ink. In a few areas, recordings may be done in red ink so they are easier to see. Pencils are not used because entries made by a pencil can be erased. Since this is a legal record, the recording must be permanent. Dots denoting measurements should be on the correct age and measurement line. A ruler or straight edge should be used to connect recordings to create the graph.

Birth to 36 months: Boys
Length-for-age and Weight-for-age percentiles

NAME Kobelak, Hayden

RECORD # 84562

AGE (MONTHS)

LENGTH

WEIGHT

LENGTH

WEIGHT

	Mother's Stature		Gestational		Comment
	Father's Stature		Age: _____ Weeks		
Date	Age	Weight	Length	Head Circ.	
3-26-02	Birth	8' 8"	19 3/4"	14 1/4"	
6-27-02	3 mo.	12' 10"	23 1/4"	15 3/4"	
9-23-02	6 mo.	17'	26"	17 1/2"	
12-20-02	9 mo.	21' 12"	28 1/2"	18 1/4"	

Published May 30, 2000 (modified 4/20/01).
SOURCE: Developed by the National Center for Health Statistics in collaboration with
the National Center for Chronic Disease Prevention and Health Promotion (2000).
http://www.cdc.gov/growthcharts

SAFER · HEALTHIER · PEOPLE™

PRACTICAL PROBLEMS

1. Kaleigh Nartker was born on July 24, —. The following are her height and weight measurements as recorded by her pediatrician. On a graph for an infant girl, age birth to 36 months, record and graph the measurements listed.

Age in Months	Length in Inches	Weight in Pounds
Birth	$20\frac{1}{2}$	$8\frac{1}{2}$
3	24	$12\frac{3}{4}$
6	$27\frac{1}{4}$	$15\frac{1}{4}$
9	29	$21\frac{1}{2}$
12	$30\frac{3}{4}$	$24\frac{1}{4}$
16	$32\frac{1}{2}$	28
23	$34\frac{1}{4}$	$32\frac{1}{2}$

2. Hayden Kobelak was born on March 15, —. The following are his height and weight measurements as recorded by his pediatrician. On a graph for an infant boy, age birth to 36 months, record and graph the measurements listed.

Age in Months	Length in Cm	Weight in Kg
Birth	48	2.8
2	52	4.2
4	59	4.8
6	64	5.6
9	67	7.2
12	73	8.6
14	76	9.4
18	81	10.2
23	86	11.8

Birth to 36 months: Girls
Length-for-age and Weight-for-age percentiles

NAME _____

RECORD # _____

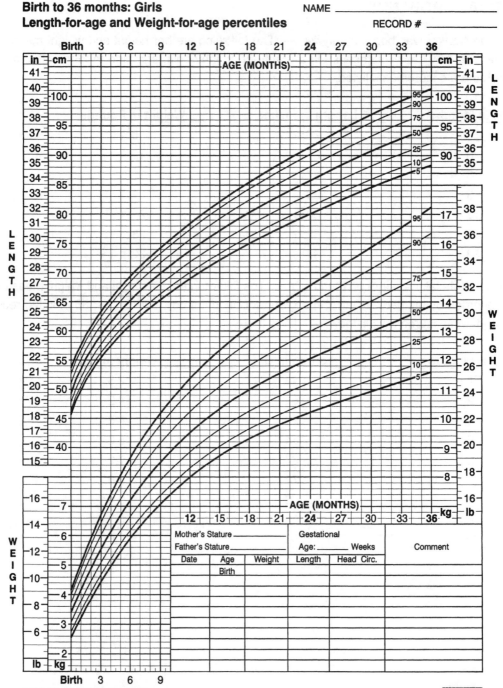

Published May 30, 2000 (modified 4/20/01).
SOURCE: Developed by the National Center for Health Statistics in collaboration with
the National Center for Chronic Disease Prevention and Health Promotion (2000).
http://www.cdc.gov/growthcharts

SAFER · HEALTHIER · PEOPLE™

Birth to 36 months: Boys
Length-for-age and Weight-for-age percentiles

NAME _____

RECORD # _____

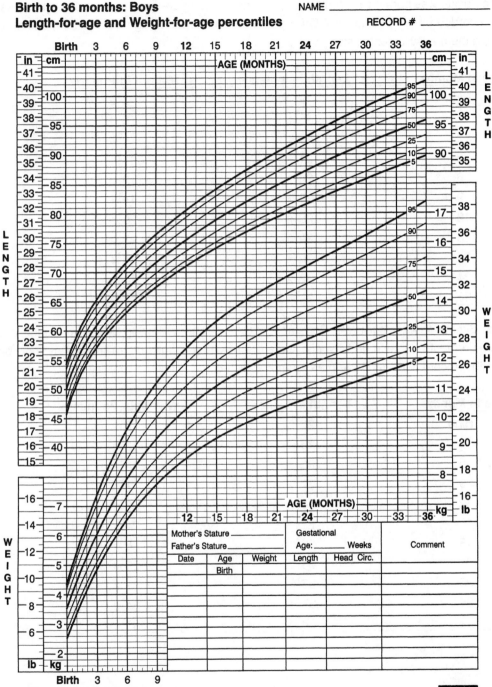

Published May 30, 2000 (modified 4/20/01).
SOURCE: Developed by the National Center for Health Statistics in collaboration with
the National Center for Chronic Disease Prevention and Health Promotion (2000).
http://www.cdc.gov/growthcharts

SAFER·HEALTHIER·PEOPLE™

3. Lisa Zucker was born on September 27, —. The following are her height and weight measurements as recorded by her pediatrician. On a graph for an infant girl, age birth to 36 months, record and graph the measurements listed.

Age in Months	Length in Inches	Weight in Pounds
Birth	$19\frac{1}{4}$	$7\frac{1}{2}$
1	$19\frac{1}{2}$	$8\frac{1}{4}$
2	$20\frac{1}{4}$	$9\frac{3}{4}$
3	$21\frac{3}{4}$	$11\frac{1}{4}$
6	$24\frac{3}{4}$	$12\frac{1}{2}$
9	$25\frac{1}{4}$	$14\frac{1}{4}$
12	$26\frac{1}{2}$	$20\frac{1}{2}$
16	29	$23\frac{1}{2}$
20	$30\frac{1}{4}$	$24\frac{3}{4}$
24	$32\frac{1}{2}$	$28\frac{1}{4}$
30	$34\frac{3}{4}$	$30\frac{1}{2}$

4. Joe Simmers was born on December 23, —. The following are his height and weight measurements as recorded by his pediatrician. On a graph for an infant boy, age birth to 36 months, record and graph the measurements listed.

Age in Months	Length in Inches	Weight in Pounds
Birth	$20\frac{1}{4}$	$9\frac{1}{2}$
3	$25\frac{1}{4}$	$12\frac{1}{4}$
6	$26\frac{1}{4}$	$14\frac{1}{2}$
9	$27\frac{1}{2}$	$17\frac{1}{4}$
12	$30\frac{1}{2}$	$20\frac{1}{2}$
15	32	$24\frac{1}{4}$
18	$33\frac{3}{4}$	$26\frac{3}{4}$
21	$34\frac{1}{2}$	$29\frac{1}{4}$
25	$35\frac{1}{4}$	$32\frac{1}{4}$
28	$37\frac{1}{4}$	$34\frac{1}{2}$
32	$38\frac{1}{2}$	$35\frac{1}{4}$

Birth to 36 months: Girls
Length-for-age and Weight-for-age percentiles

NAME _____

RECORD # _____

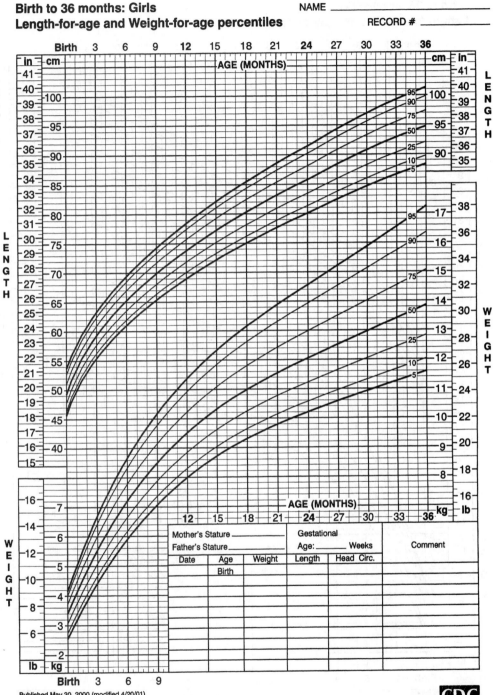

Published May 30, 2000 (modified 4/20/01).
SOURCE: Developed by the National Center for Health Statistics in collaboration with
the National Center for Chronic Disease Prevention and Health Promotion (2000).
http://www.cdc.gov/growthcharts

SAFER · HEALTHIER · PEOPLE™

Birth to 36 months: Boys
Length-for-age and Weight-for-age percentiles

NAME _____

RECORD # _____

AGE (MONTHS)

Birth 3 6 9 12 15 18 21 24 27 30 33 36

LENGTH

WEIGHT

AGE (MONTHS)

| | 12 | 15 | 18 | 21 | 24 | 27 | 30 | 33 | 36 | kg | lb |

Mother's Stature _____

Father's Stature _____

Gestational
Age: _____ Weeks

Comment

Date	Age	Weight	Length	Head Circ.
	Birth			

Birth 3 6 9

Published May 30, 2000 (modified 4/20/01).
SOURCE: Developed by the National Center for Health Statistics in collaboration with
the National Center for Chronic Disease Prevention and Health Promotion (2000).
http://www.cdc.gov/growthcharts

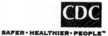

SAFER · HEALTHIER · PEOPLE™

5. Gina Ashley was born prematurely on February 27, —. The following are her height and weight measurements as recorded by her pediatrician. On a graph for an infant girl, age birth to 36 months, record and graph the measurements listed.

Age in Months	Length in Centimeters	Weight in Kilograms
Birth	40	1.8
1	43	2.4
2	45.5	3.2
3	47	3.8
4	51	4.6
5	55	5.6
6	59	6
8	64.5	6.8
10	68	8
12	72	8.6
15	74	9.4
19	78	10.6
22	81	10.8
25	85	11.5
30	90	12.4

6. Dick Szabo was born on October 11, —. The following are his height and weight measurements as recorded by his pediatrician. On a graph for an infant boy, age birth to 36 months, record and graph the measurements listed.

Age in Months	Length in Centimeters	Weight in Kilograms
Birth	55	4.4
1	60	5
3	64.5	6.8
6	70	9.2
9	75	10.8
12	80	12.2
16	83	12.8
19	86.5	13.6
22	88	14.5
26	91	15.2
30	97	15.8
34	99	16.6

Birth to 36 months: Girls
Length-for-age and Weight-for-age percentiles

NAME _____

RECORD # _____

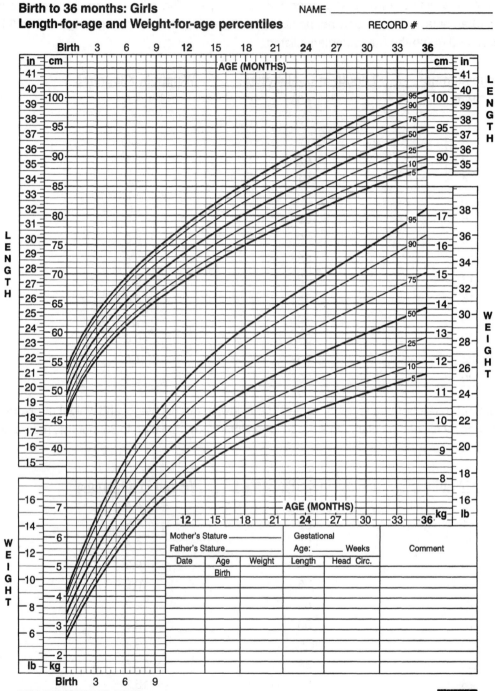

Published May 30, 2000 (modified 4/20/01).
SOURCE: Developed by the National Center for Health Statistics in collaboration with
the National Center for Chronic Disease Prevention and Health Promotion (2000).
http://www.cdc.gov/growthcharts

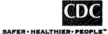

SAFER · HEALTHIER · PEOPLE™

Birth to 36 months: Boys
Length-for-age and Weight-for-age percentiles

NAME _____

RECORD # _____

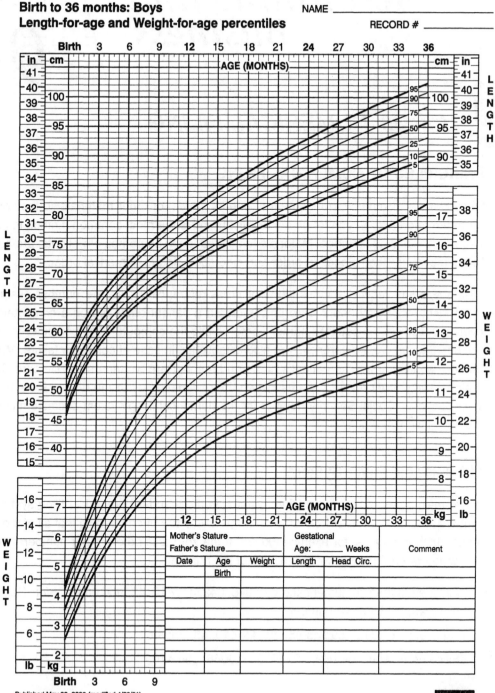

AGE (MONTHS)

Mother's Stature _____
Father's Stature _____

Gestational
Age: _____ Weeks

Comment

Date	Age	Weight	Length	Head Circ.
	Birth			

Published May 30, 2000 (modified 4/20/01).
SOURCE: Developed by the National Center for Health Statistics in collaboration with
the National Center for Chronic Disease Prevention and Health Promotion (2000).
http://www.cdc.gov/growthcharts

SAFER·HEALTHIER·PEOPLE™

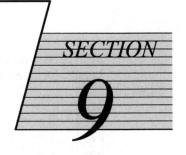

Accounting and Business

Unit 38 NUMERICAL FILING

BASIC PRINCIPLES OF NUMERICAL FILING

Filing is the systematic or orderly arrangement of papers, cards, or other materials so they are readily available for future reference. Even though alphabetical filing is the most common method in use, many agencies use numerical filing methods. Materials to be filed, such as names of patients, are assigned a number. The numbers are then placed in order and filed according to numerical order.

Numerical filing systems require a cross-index or cross-reference list so the number assigned to a patient can be identified. Many health care offices create a patient database on a computer. When a patient arrives at the office, the patient's name is entered into the computer. The computer then lists the patient's number. Backup cross-references are also established in case of computer failure. Many of the backup systems use file cards. The patient's name and number are written on the file card. The cards are filed in alphabetical order for easy access when the patient comes to the office. Some health care agencies use a patient's Social Security number for the numerical filing system because most patients know their Social Security number.

Standard Numerical Filing System:

One of the two main types of numerical filing systems is the standard numerical filing system. In this system, numbers always go in order from small to large. Zeros are often used so that all of the numbers have the same number of digits, for example 00235. If the zero falls before other numbers, the zero is usually disregarded when filing, but written in front of the number.

Example: File the numbers in numerical order: 045, 042, 44, 410, 43, and 0046. (*Hint:* Remember to disregard "0" before a number.)

Numbers would be read as 45, 42, 44, 410, 43, and 46

Filing order would be 042, 43, 44, 045, 0046, and 410

Terminal Digit Filing System:

The second main type of numerical filing system is the terminal or last digit filing system. In this type of system, the last digits are used to group or file records. For example, one series of charts may contain 24 as the last digits and another series of charts may contain 28 as the last digits. The series of charts ending in 24 would be filed as one group, and the series of charts ending in 28 would be filed as a separate group.

Example: File the numbers in numerical order using the terminal digit numerical system: 01-654-28, 09-523-24, 07-733-24, 08-569-24, 23-411-28, 03-891-24, 00-678-28, and 23-408-28

First separate the numbers into two systems based on the terminal digits:

01-654-28, 23-411-28, 00-678-28, and 23-408-28

09-523-24, 07-733-24, 08-569-24, and 03-891-24

Next put each system in correct filing order:

00-678-28, 01-654-28, 23-408-28, and 23-411-28

03-891-24, 07-733-24, 08-569-24, and 09-523-24

Now put the systems in order. Since the digit 24 precedes 28, the terminal system with 24 is placed first:

03-891-24, 07-733-24, 08-569-24, and 09-523-24

00-678-28, 01-654-28, 23-408-28, and 23-411-28

PRACTICAL PROBLEMS

1.   Put the following numbers in numerical order: 23, 904, 831, 567, 25, 829, 554, 523, 22, and 568.

_____   _____   _____   _____   _____

_____   _____   _____   _____   _____

2.   Put the following numbers in numerical order: 0234, 0345, 0956, 0487, 0390, 0475, 0948, 0324, 0253, 0354, 0221, 0495, 0233, 0965, and 0389.

_____   _____   _____   _____   _____

_____   _____   _____   _____   _____

_____   _____   _____   _____   _____

3. Put the following numbers in numerical order: 88-93, 78-92, 08-94, 07-56, 71-52, 00-56, 02-92, 88-94, 71-25, 78-25, 02-94, 88-92, 88-25, 71-92, and 08-92.

    _____   _____   _____   _____   _____

    _____   _____   _____   _____   _____

    _____   _____   _____   _____   _____

4. Put the following numbers in numerical order: 00289, 0567, 234, 5009, 900, 8602, 034, 000235, 2870, and 0233.

    _____   _____   _____   _____   _____

    _____   _____   _____   _____   _____

5. Put the following numbers in numerical order: 50, 555, 0543, 055, 05, 500, 511, 056, 00571, 00553, 0000556, 05000, 051, 00510, and 05011.

    _____   _____   _____   _____   _____

    _____   _____   _____   _____   _____

    _____   _____   _____   _____   _____

6. Put the following numbers in order using the terminal digit system: 89-30, 89-29, 76-30, 85-29, 75-30, 86-30, 76-29, 87-29, 84-30, and 75-29.

    System 1:

    _____   _____   _____   _____   _____

    System 2:

    _____   _____   _____   _____   _____

7. Put the following numbers in order using the terminal digit system: 32-41-65, 32-40-55, 65-65-65, 56-41-55, 65-40-65, 65-41-55, 32-40-65, 33-40-55, 65-40-55, and 64-41-65.

    System 1:

    _____   _____   _____   _____   _____

    System 2:

    _____   _____   _____   _____   _____

8. Put the following numbers in order using the terminal digit system: 0894-98, 0895-99, 00889-99, 893-98, 00891-98, 0899-99, 000891-99, 897-99, 00890-98, 000889-98, 895-98, and 00892-99.

   System 1:

   _____   _____   _____

   _____   _____   _____

   System 2:

   _____   _____   _____

   _____   _____   _____

9. Put the following numbers in order using the terminal digit system: 0340-111, 341-110, 3440-110, 03401-111, 034-111, 3400-111, 34-110, 000341-111, 03041-111, 3401-110, 003441-110, and 00314-110.

   System 1:

   _____   _____   _____

   _____   _____   _____

   System 2:

   _____   _____   _____

   _____   _____   _____

10. Put the following numbers in order using the terminal digit system: 098-7555-654, 0894-41-656, 0000-890-654, 987-52-654, 9854-656, 0895-4-654, 00890-14-654, 0895-00-656, 85941-0-656, 000-891-4-656, 008-50-9422-656, 000890-15-654, 00987-576-654, 0098-7520-654, 0009-87-654, 00850-9420-656, 08-5094-21-656, and 0000-891-656.

System 1:

_____   _____   _____

_____   _____   _____

_____   _____   _____

System 2:

_____   _____   _____

_____   _____   _____

_____   _____   _____

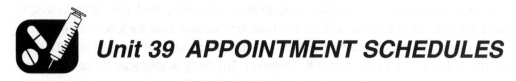

Unit 39 APPOINTMENT SCHEDULES

BASIC PRINCIPLES OF SCHEDULING APPOINTMENTS

Scheduling appointments efficiently is important in any health care facility. If done correctly, it eliminates long waiting times for patients and unscheduled time for health care personnel. In many health care agencies, appointment scheduling is done by computer. The computer automatically locates the next available time and date, provides a record of appointments already scheduled, can be programmed to schedule a set block of time for a particular procedure, and prints out copies of the daily schedule. Most software used for appointment scheduling is user-friendly and easy to use. However, it is still important to understand the basic principles behind scheduling appointments. Computerized scheduling can be efficient and convenient, but an alternate system must exist for downtime, or times when the computer is not functioning correctly. Manual scheduling of appointments involves the use of appointment books.

Appointment books vary from office to office. Most contain one or one-half page for each day. Time is usually blocked off in quarter-hour periods. It is essential that the person scheduling knows what block of time each line represents.

DATE:		DATE: Tuesday, 6/23/—	
8:30 ↓	8:30 to 8:45	8:30	(Office Meeting)
8:45 ↓	8:45 to 9:00	8:45	
9:00 ↓	9:00 to 9:15	9:00	
9:15 ↓	9:15 to 9:30	9:15	
9:30 ↓	15 minutes	9:30 ↓	Matt Kiser - BP Check
9:45	30 minutes	9:45	Dennis Bartlett -
10:00 ↓		10:00 ↓	Tumor Removal
10:15	45 minutes	10:15	Sharon Townsend -
10:30		10:30	Toenail Surgery
10:45 ↓		10:45 ↓	
11:00	60 minutes or	11:00	Brian Bowen - Physical
11:15	1 hour	11:15	
11:30		11:30	
11:45 ↓		11:45 ↓	

In the example appointment schedule shown, the left-hand column is marked with the time periods represented. Each line equals a 15-minute block of time. If an appointment takes longer than 15 minutes, an arrow is drawn to indicate the time period needed. Study the examples shown for a 15-, 30-, 45-, and 60-minute period of time. In the right-hand column, patients are scheduled for the blocks of time shown in the left-hand column. Most agencies block out periods of time when the individual for whom appointments are being scheduled is not available. An example is shown by the large "X" from 8:30 to 9:30 in the right-hand column. Other examples of blocked-out time include time for lunch, meetings, or afternoons off. Note that the blocked-out time for the 8:30 to 9:30 meeting ends at the 9:15 line. This line represents the time from 9:15 to 9:30, or the end of the meeting. The first line available for appointments would be the 9:30 line since this represents the time from 9:30 to 9:45. Remember this time sequence while completing the practical problems on scheduling appointments.

PRACTICAL PROBLEMS

1. You are employed in a dental office as a receptionist. Use the appointment schedule to record the following appointments.

    a. In the date column, print Monday and a date on the top of one column. Print Tuesday and the next day's date at the top of the second column.

    b. Block out lunch periods which are from 12:00 to 1:00 each day. (*Hint:* Remember lunch ends at 1:00.)

    c. The doctor has a Dental Board Meeting from 8:30 to 10:00 on Tuesday morning. Block out this period of time.

    d. Ed Holmes calls for an appointment to replace an amalgam restoration (Amal). He prefers a 1:00 appointment on Tuesday. It will take 30 minutes.

    e. Carol Martin needs an appointment for a prophylactic (Prophy) cleaning and fluoride (Fl) treatment. She prefers early Monday morning and requires 45 minutes.

    f. Karen Carey needs an appointment for a fitting on a crown (Cr). She prefers early Monday afternoon and requires 15 minutes.

    g. Jerry Beal must have a wisdom tooth extracted (Ext). He prefers early Monday morning and requires 30 minutes.

    h. Linda Knowlton needs a composite restoration (Comp). She prefers early afternoon on Monday and requires 45 minutes.

    i. Tom Grandy needs a prophylactic (Prophy) cleaning and exam (Ex). He will require 45 minutes and prefers late Tuesday morning.

    j. Penny Sheely needs an appointment for her two children, Mike and Mark, for an exam (Ex) and fluoride (Fl) treatment. Each child will require 15 minutes and she prefers early Tuesday morning.

    k. Tom Tenney needs endodontic (Endo) work that will require 1½ hours. He prefers a Tuesday afternoon appointment.

    l. Joyce Feltner needs a composite (Comp) restoration that will require 30 minutes. She prefers Monday morning.

m. Jackie Frank needs a 45-minute appointment for a crown (Cr) replacement. She prefers Monday afternoon.

n. Tom Wolf needs a 45-minute appointment for a prophylactic (Prophy) cleaning and exam (Ex). He prefers Monday morning.

o. Dave Berry needs an amalgam (Amal) restoration. This will require 30 minutes and he prefers Tuesday afternoon.

p. Shelly Barr needs an hour appointment for an endodontic (Endo) treatment. She prefers Monday morning.

q. Pam Mock needs an appointment for her three children for a prophylactic (Prophy) cleaning and fluoride (Fl) treatment. Tom will require 30 minutes, and Trevor and Tim will require 15 minutes each. She prefers Tuesday afternoon.

r. Phil Bush needs a 30-minute appointment for an amalgam (Amal) restoration. He prefers Monday afternoon.

s. Kelly Purvis needs a composite (Comp) restoration that will require 30 minutes. She prefers Tuesday morning.

t. Kathy Schultheis needs two wisdom teeth extracted (Ext). This will require $1\frac{1}{4}$ hours. She can come in either Monday or Tuesday afternoon.

u. Nancy Darbey needs bite-wing X rays (BWXR). They will take 15 minutes and she prefers a morning appointment.

v. Randal Cooper needs a crown (Cr) reattached. He will require 15 minutes and can come in anytime on Monday.

APPOINTMENT SCHEDULE

DATE:	DATE:
8:30	8:30
8:45	8:45
9:00	9:00
9:15	9:15
9:30	9:30
9:45	9:45
10:00	10:00
10:15	10:15
10:30	10:30
10:45	10:45
11:00	11:00
11:15	11:15
11:30	11:30
11:45	11:45
12:00	12:00
12:15	12:15
12:30	12:30
12:45	12:45
1:00	1:00
1:15	1:15
1:30	1:30
1:45	1:45
2:00	2:00
2:15	2:15
2:30	2:30
2:45	2:45
3:00	3:00
3:15	3:15
3:30	3:30
3:45	3:45
4:00	4:00
4:15	4:15
4:30	4:30

2. You are employed in a medical office. Use the appointment schedule to record the following appointments.

    a. In the date column, print Wednesday and a date at the top of one column. Print Thursday and the next day's date at the top of the second column.

    b. The physician is not in the office until 9:00 A.M. because she makes hospital rounds in the morning. Lunch is scheduled from 12 Noon until 1:00 P.M.

    c. On Thursday, the physician has a medical board meeting at the hospital from 12:30 until 2:30 P.M. She will return to the office by 3:00 P.M.

    d. Mrs. Eleanor Probasco (Gene) wants an appointment for a physical examination on Thursday afternoon. The physical will take one hour.

    e. Mr. Jim Marcinko needs an appointment for an allergy shot early Wednesday morning. The nurse gives the injection and the patient does *not* have to see the physician. The injection will require 15 minutes.

    f. Mrs. Karen Nartker (Brian) needs an appointment for her triplets, Mike, Paul, and Steve. They need immunization injections. Each child will take 10 minutes. She prefers an early appointment on Wednesday afternoon.

    g. Mrs. Margo Thayer (Bob) needs an early appointment Wednesday morning to have a wart removed from her foot. This will take about one-half hour.

    h. Mrs. Carol Lake (Jim) wants an appointment for 9:45 Thursday morning. She has a severe upper respiratory infection (URI). The appointment should require 15 minutes.

    i. Mrs. Sharon Logan (Tom) needs an appointment Thursday morning for a Pap test. This requires 15 minutes.

    j. Anna Herb calls and wants an appointment for a physical examination early on Thursday morning. This will require one hour.

    k. Linda Butcher calls and wants an early appointment on Wednesday. She has laryngitis. This will require 15 minutes.

    l. Mrs. Jane Baker (Lee) would like an appointment Wednesday morning for surgery on her fractured toe. This should require 45 minutes.

    m. Peggy Montagno needs an appointment on Wednesday morning. She has an ear infection. This will require 15 minutes.

    n. Mrs. Diane Morrison (Bob) would like an appointment late Thursday morning for a physical examination. This will require one hour.

    o. Mrs. Sharon Kobelak (Mike) needs an appointment for her four children. They all have colds. She prefers Wednesday at 2:00 P.M. Each child will require about 10 minutes.

    p. Mrs. Debbie Benevento (Duke) needs an appointment Wednesday morning to have a growth removed from her right arm. The surgery will require one hour.

q. Pam Bauerle has a skin rash and has decided to have allergy tests. She prefers a Thursday morning appointment. The tests will take approximately one-half hour.

r. John Wheaton needs an appointment for a chest X ray. He also has a severe cough. He prefers 4:00 P.M. on Thursday. The procedure will take about 30 minutes.

s. Pam Cook would like an appointment for a physical examination. She can come anytime after 2 P.M. on Wednesday. The examination will take one hour.

t. Mrs. Marilyn Weiss (Gary) has stomach cramps. She also needs a review of her current medications. She can come anytime after 3:00 P.M. Wednesday. The examination will take about 30 minutes.

u. Floyd Simmons needs an appointment for a repeat X ray on his fractured arm. He can come anytime Wednesday afternoon. The X ray will take about 15 minutes.

v. Steve Drapach needs an appointment for allergy shots. He must be seen by the physician. He prefers early Wednesday afternoon. The shots will take 15 minutes.

w. Mrs. Pat Reno (Tom) needs an appointment to check her blood pressure. This will take about $\frac{1}{4}$ hour. She prefers Wednesday afternoon.

APPOINTMENT SCHEDULE

DATE:	DATE:
8:30	8:30
8:45	8:45
9:00	9:00
9:15	9:15
9:30	9:30
9:45	9:45
10:00	10:00
10:15	10:15
10:30	10:30
10:45	10:45
11:00	11:00
11:15	11:15
11:30	11:30
11:45	11:45
12:00	12:00
12:15	12:15
12:30	12:30
12:45	12:45
1:00	1:00
1:15	1:15
1:30	1:30
1:45	1:45
2:00	2:00
2:15	2:15
2:30	2:30
2:45	2:45
3:00	3:00
3:15	3:15
3:30	3:30
3:45	3:45
4:00	4:00
4:15	4:15
4:30	4:30

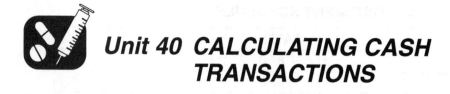

Unit 40 CALCULATING CASH TRANSACTIONS

BASIC PRINCIPLES OF CALCULATING CASH TRANSACTIONS

Cash transactions occur in most health care agencies. Proper handling of these transactions is essential. Most agencies maintain a cash drawer that contains currency and coins. When a patient or client pays a bill in cash, the correct amount of change must be given to the patient from the cash drawer. At the end of the day, the amounts must balance.

The easiest way to calculate change due the patient is to subtract the amount of the bill from the cash amount given by the patient. If a bill is $26.50, and a patient pays with two twenty-dollar bills or $40, subtract $26.50 from $40 to get $13.50 change due the patient. Then calculate how to give $13.50 with the least amount of coins and currency. One ten-dollar bill, three one-dollar bills, and two quarters will equal $13.50. While giving the change to the patient, count out the amount starting with the amount of the bill.

Example:

Say the amount of the bill:	$26.50
Give $0.25 (1 quarter) and say:	$26.75
Give $0.25 (1 quarter) and say:	$27.00
Give $1 bill and say:	$28.00
Give $1 bill and say:	$29.00
Give $10 bill and say:	$40.00

It is always best to keep the amount given by the patient separate or turned sideways in the cash drawer until the change has been given. If the patient questions the amount of change and says he or she gave a different amount, for example $50, the money is still separate from other currency in the cash drawer and can be used to verify the amount given. When currency is placed in the cash drawer, keep each denomination of currency in its own area or compartment in the drawer. It is also best to turn all of the bills face up and in the same direction. This prevents using a $10 bill when a $1 bill is needed. Coins should also be separated by type into individual compartments.

At the end of the day, the cash drawer should balance. Many agencies use a balance sheet for this purpose. Each type of coin and currency is added together to determine the total balance in the cash drawer. The amount of money in the cash drawer at the start of the day is added to the cash payments received during the day. If money in the cash drawer was used to pay a bill, this amount is subtracted to obtain the final balance that should be in the cash drawer. Study the sample balance sheet.

DAILY CASH DRAWER BALANCE SHEET

Date: _____ July 29, 20— _____

NUMBER	DENOMINATION		AMOUNT
28	Pennies	(× .01)	.28
31	Nickels	(× .05)	1.55
28	Dimes	(× .10)	2.80
43	Quarters	(× .25)	10.75
0	Half-Dollars	(× .50)	0.00
84	$1 Bills	(× 1.00)	84.00
23	$5 Bills	(× 5.00)	115.00
19	$10 Bills	(× 10.00)	190.00
16	$20 Bills	(× 20.00)	320.00
5	$50 Bills	(× 50.00)	250.00
3	$100 Bills	(× 100.00)	300.00
	TOTAL AMOUNT		1274.38

Beginning Cash Balance	40.00
+ Total of Cash Payments	1259.63
TOTAL	1299.63
- Payments Made from Cash Drawer	25.25
FINAL CASH AMOUNT	1274.38

Every denomination of coins and currency was counted and the number of each was noted in the left-hand column under "Number." The number was then multiplied by the value for the denomination, shown in parentheses, and the value or amount put in the right-hand column. All amounts were added to obtain the total amount in the cash drawer. The balance at the bottom shows a $40.00 beginning cash balance in the drawer at the start of the day. This is added to the total of cash payments made during the day. The amount of $25.25 was paid out of the cash drawer so it is subtracted from the total. Since the "Final Cash Amount" equals the "Total Amount," the cash drawer balances for the day.

PRACTICAL PROBLEMS

For problems 1 to 10, list the amount of money given to the patient in change starting with the amount of the bill.

1.   The patient's bill is $32 and the patient pays with a $50 bill.

                                 Say _____

Give _____   Say _____

Give _____   Say _____

Give _____   Say _____

Give _____   Say _____

Give _____   Say _____

2.   The patient's bill is $54.50 and the patient pays with three $20 bills.

                                 Say _____

Give _____   Say _____

Give _____   Say _____

Give _____   Say _____

3.   The patient's bill is $12.65 and the patient pays with a $10 bill and a $5 bill.

                                 Say _____

Give _____   Say _____

Give _____   Say _____

Give _____   Say _____

Give _____   Say _____

4.   The patient's bill is $31.75 and the patient pays with a $50 bill.

                                 Say _____

Give _____   Say _____

Give _____   Say _____

Give _____   Say _____

Give _____   Say _____

Give _____   Say _____

Give _____   Say _____

5.   The patient's bill is $65.85 and the patient pays with a $100 bill.

Say _____

Give _____   Say _____

Give _____   Say _____

Give _____   Say _____

Give _____   Say _____

Give _____   Say _____

Give _____   Say _____

Give _____   Say _____

Give _____   Say _____

6.   The patient's bill is $25.09 and the patient pays with two $20 bills.

Say _____

Give _____   Say _____

Give _____   Say _____

Give _____   Say _____

Give _____   Say _____

Give _____   Say _____

Give _____   Say _____

Give _____   Say _____

Give _____   Say _____

Give _____   Say _____

Give _____   Say _____

Give _____   Say _____

7.   The patient's bill is $43.58 and the patient pays with three $20 bills.

Say _____

Give _____   Say _____

Give _____   Say _____

Give _____   Say _____

Give _____   Say _____

Give _____   Say _____

Give _____   Say _____

Give _____   Say _____

Give _____   Say _____

8.   The patient's bill is $24.50. The patient also has a previous balance due for $32.75 and wants to pay the total bill. The patient pays with a $50 bill and a $20 bill.

                          Say _____

Give _____   Say _____

Give _____   Say _____

Give _____   Say _____

Give _____   Say _____

Give _____   Say _____

Give _____   Say _____

9.   The patient is paying for two children. One bill is $64.35 and the second bill is $41.20. The patient pays with one $50 bill and three $20 bills.

                          Say _____

Give _____   Say _____

Give _____   Say _____

Give _____   Say _____

Give _____   Say _____

Give _____   Say _____

Give _____   Say _____

Give _____   Say _____

10. The patient's bill is $71.20 and the patient pays with one quarter, a $50 bill, a $20 bill, and a $10 bill.

                          Say _____

Give _____   Say _____

Give _____   Say _____

Give _____   Say _____

Give _____   Say _____

Give _____   Say _____

Give _____   Say _____

DAILY CASH DRAWER BALANCE SHEET

Date: _____ 10 / 11 / —_____

NUMBER	DENOMINATION		AMOUNT
45	Pennies	(× .01)	
132	Nickels	(× .05)	
92	Dimes	(× .10)	
136	Quarters	(× .25)	
7	Half-Dollars	(× .50)	
61	$1 Bills	(× 1.00)	
22	$5 Bills	(× 5.00)	
18	$10 Bills	(× 10.00)	
12	$20 Bills	(× 20.00)	
3	$50 Bills	(× 50.00)	
2	$100 Bills	(× 100.00)	
	TOTAL AMOUNT		

Beginning Cash Balance	
+ Total of Cash Payments	
TOTAL	
- Payments Made from Cash Drawer	
FINAL CASH AMOUNT	

11. Use the *Daily Cash Drawer Balance Sheet* to calculate the amount shown in the cash drawer. There was $50 in the cash drawer at the start of the day. Total cash payments received for the day were $944.75. No payments were made from the cash drawer.

   a. What is the total amount in the cash drawer? _____

   b. Does the final cash amount equal the right amount? If not, how much over or under is the balance? _____

DAILY CASH DRAWER BALANCE SHEET

Date: _____ 10 / 12 / — _____

NUMBER	DENOMINATION		AMOUNT
98	Pennies	(× .01)	
89	Nickels	(× .05)	
109	Dimes	(× .10)	
161	Quarters	(× .25)	
12	Half-Dollars	(× .50)	
329	$1 Bills	(× 1.00)	
77	$5 Bills	(× 5.00)	
68	$10 Bills	(× 10.00)	
81	$20 Bills	(× 20.00)	
11	$50 Bills	(× 50.00)	
3	$100 Bills	(× 100.00)	
	TOTAL AMOUNT		

Beginning Cash Balance	
+ Total of Cash Payments	
TOTAL	
- Payments Made from Cash Drawer	
FINAL CASH AMOUNT	

12. Use the *Daily Cash Drawer Balance Sheet* to calculate the amount shown in the cash drawer. There was $30 in the cash drawer at the start of the day. Total cash payments received for the day were $4,139.45. The amount spent from the cash drawer was $242.95.

   a. What is the total amount in the cash drawer?   _____

   b. Does the final cash amount equal the right amount? If not, how much over or under is the balance?   _____

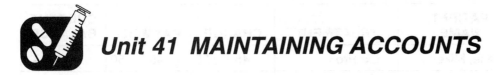

Unit 41 MAINTAINING ACCOUNTS

BASIC PRINCIPLES OF MAINTAINING ACCOUNTS

Maintaining accounts accurately is an essential part of any health care field. An *account* can be defined as a financial record of charges, payments made, and amounts due. A *charge* is a fee charged for a service. A *payment* is an amount of money paid by a patient or client. A *current balance* is the amount still owed by the patient or client and is often classified as accounts receivable.

Many health care agencies use computerized bookkeeping systems. Most systems used begin with the creation of a patient's account history. Information including the name and address of the patient, the person responsible for paying the account, family members in the account, and insurance information is entered for each patient. This forms the data base of the computerized system. Procedures performed in the health care agency are programmed into the computer along with insurance procedure codes and fees charged for each procedure. Most software is also programmed to indicate a source of payment, such as cash, check, or insurance payment. When a patient receives a service, the patient's account history is retrieved. The service provided is entered into the computer, usually by procedure code number. The software in the computer automatically calculates the current balance by using the past balance in the account history and adding it to the new charges. If payment is made, the software deducts the payment and calculates the new current balance. The account history is updated automatically as entries are made. Printed copies of the account can be given to the patient to show all charges, payments made, and current balance due. In addition, the account history can be printed and mailed to the patient as a monthly bill. Most software programs will also create a daily journal that provides a complete financial record showing patients seen, services provided, charges, payments made, and outstanding balances (or accounts receivable). In addition, many programs will create a daily deposit slip for all payments made during the day. This can be used to deposit the monies received (cash and checks) in the bank at the end of the day.

Most computerized billing systems are easy to use. However, safeguards must be in place to protect the financial information. Most agencies use password protection so only authorized individuals are allowed access to the information. The system must also be programmed to record deleted transactions to prevent someone from deleting a transaction and stealing the money. Daily tape, disk, or CD-ROM backups must be made of all information and stored in a safe area in case of computer failure.

Even though computerized systems can calculate financial transactions, the health care worker must still understand the basic principles of billing. Even computers can make mistakes. In addition, if computer failure occurs, the agency must still have access to financial information. For this reason, most health care agencies use printed copies of some type of ledger card to keep a record of financial transactions.

DATE	PATIENT NAME	TREATMENT	CHARGE		PAYMENT		CURRENT BALANCE	
8/14	Base, Mike	Ex, Pro	45	50	45	50	—	—
8/26	Base, Mike	Amalgam	52	50	45	00	7	50
8/30	Base, Mike	Endodontics	77	25	50	00	34	75
9/8	Base, Mike	Crown	96	00	28	00	102	75
9/26	Base, Mike	ROA-Insur.	—	—	95	00	7	75

In the sample ledger card shown, the date, patient's name, and the treatment given are shown in the first three columns. The fourth column shows the charge for the treatment. Payment made by the patient is recorded in the fifth column. The payment made is subtracted from the charge to equal the current balance. In the first example, payment is made in full so there is no current balance. If a current balance exists, this becomes a previous balance when a new charge is noted. The following formula is used to calculate current balance:

Previous Balance + Charge − Payment = Current Balance

On the second line of the sample ledger card, a current balance of $7.50 is present. This becomes a previous balance and is added to the charge on line three before payment is subtracted.

Example: Previous Balance (line 2) = $7.50   Charge (line 3) = $77.25

Previous Balance + Charge = Balance Due $7.50 + 77.25 = $84.75

Balance Due − Payment = Current Balance $84.75 − 50.00 = $34.75

If the current balance on the ledger card is not added to the charge, this amount of money due would be lost and the account would not balance. At times, payment is received without a charge being made. The fifth line of the sample ledger shows a payment received on account from an insurance company. Since this is not a treatment, no charge is noted. The current balance becomes the previous balance of $102.75 on the fourth line. The payment of $95.00 is subtracted from the $102.75 to give a current balance due of $7.75. In many agencies, a copy of the ledger card is mailed to the patient as a bill. The patient is told to pay the last amount in the current balance column.

PRACTICAL PROBLEMS

1. A new patient has no previous balance. He is treated for a burn with a charge of $44 and pays $20. What is his current balance? _____

2. A patient with a current balance of $135.96 visits the office. She is treated for bronchitis with a charge of $57.50. She pays $32.00. What is her new current balance? _____

3. An insurance company sends a payment for $640.25 on an account that has a current balance of $842.36. What is the new current balance of the account? _____

4. A dental patient with a current balance of $137.40 on her account has an examination with a charge of $45.50, a fluoride treatment with a charge of $28.50, and four bite-wing X rays with a charge of $52.80. She makes no payment. What is her new current balance? _____

5. A family has a current balance of $106.25 when the parents bring their three children to a dental office. All three children have their teeth cleaned and fluoride treatments. The charge for a cleaning is $56.75 and the charge for a fluoride treatment is $28.95 The family pays $201.75. What is the new current balance? _____

6. A patient with a current balance of $78.32 is treated for pneumonia. A chest X ray costs $126, a sputum specimen costs $62.95, an office visit costs $66.50, and medications total $93.85. He pays $155.00. What is his new current balance? _____

7. A patient has an appendectomy. Operating room charges are $2,186.00, anesthesia is $954.80, charge for a hospital room for three days is $572.42 per day, medications total $897.59, and miscellaneous charges are $739.15. The insurance company pays $5,195.84.

   a. What is the balance the patient must pay? _____

   b. What percent of the bill was paid by insurance? _____

8. A patient with a current balance of $71.23 has a physical examination for a charge of $246.40, an ECG for a charge of $124.75, blood tests for a charge of $218.45, and urine tests for a charge of $93.30. She pays $225.00. What is her new current balance? _____

9. A patient with a current balance of $231.30 has blood work done including a complete blood count (CBC) for $86.30, a fasting blood sugar (FBS) for $64.60, a hemoglobin (hgb) for $39.55, and an erythrocyte sedimentation rate (ESR) for $71.20. He pays $75.00 and his insurance company pays $196.24. What is his new current balance?   _____

10. Treatment for a fractured arm includes charges for an X ray of $106.28, cast for $374.85, 5 office visits at $55.25 each, 4 physical therapy treatments for $87.38 each, and medications at a cost of $101.19. The patient has a previous balance of $72.94. The insurance company pays 80% of the current charges and the patient pays $120.00. What is the new current balance? (*Hint:* The insurance company does not pay any amount on the previous balance.)   _____

11. A patient with a previous balance of $321.28 injures his back. A physical therapist provides a series of treatments including 4 heat pack treatments at a cost of $42.55 each, 2 whirlpool treatments at a cost of $58.40 each, 5 traction treatments at $38.95 each, 3 massage treatments for ½ hour each at a cost of $64.00 per hour, and 2 sessions of range-of-motion (ROM) exercises at $74.25 each. The insurance company pays 75% of the current charges and the patient pays a total of $355.75. What is the new current balance?   _____

12. An infant is born prematurely. The hospital charges $878.52 per day for 9 days in the premature infant nursery, $55.28 each for 8 blood tests, and $26.38 daily for oxygen supplies for each day of hospitalization. In addition, a change of $42.54 is made for each tube feeding. The first three days the infant is given a tube feeding q2h (every 2 hours), on days 4 to 5 the infant is given a tube feeding q3h (every 3 hours), and on day 6 the infant is given two tube feedings to supplement the bottle feedings. The insurance company pays 65% of all charges. The hospital allows the parents to pay the balance due with equal monthly payments for a one-year period. What is the monthly payment the parents will have to make?   _____

13. Use the ledger card to record the following medical charges and payments for Sue Steidl. She has no current balance.

3/25/–   Office visit: $68.50
           Payment of $25.00

4/14/–   Office visit: $52.45, Blood tests: $73.45
           Payment of $35.50

5/28/–   Office visit: $58.50, ECG: $112.75
           Payment of $48.50

6/2/–   Office visit: $61.30, Medications: $74.38
           No payment made

6/9/–   Insurance payment of $356.37

DATE	PATIENT NAME	TREATMENT	CHARGE	PAYMENT	CURRENT BALANCE

14. Use the ledger card to record the following dental charges and payments for Dave Baker. He has no current balance.

1/3/–	Exam and prophy treatment: $93.90
	Full mouth X-ray series: $206.65
	Payment of $95.00

| 1/14/– | 2 amalgam restorations at $48.33 each |
| | No payment made |

| 1/21/– | Insurance payment of $242.37 |

2/16/–	Rubber base impression: $34.90
	Crown preparation: $312.20
	Payment of $105.00

2/23/–	Charges for crown: $529.45
	Crown placement: $72.80
	Payment of $155.50

DATE	PATIENT NAME	TREATMENT	CHARGE		PAYMENT		CURRENT BALANCE	

15. Use the ledger card to record the following chiropractic charges and payments for Pat Lictner. She has a current balance of $586.33.

10/11/–	Spinal X rays: 4 at $42.75 each
	Spinal manipulation: ½-hour treatment at $64.50 per hour
	Payment of $25.50

| 10/19/– | Spinal manipulation: ¾-hour treatment |
| | Payment of $25.50 |

11/2/–	Acupuncture treatment: 30 minutes at $84.60 per hour
	Spinal X rays: 2 at $42.75 each
	Payment of $34.75

11/8/–	Alternate hot and cold pack treatment: $41.70
	Spinal manipulation: 15-minute treatment
	No payment made

| 11/10/– | Insurance payment ROA (received on account): $428.64 |

11/16/–	Spinal manipulation: 45-minute treatment
	Acupuncture: 20-minute treatment
	Payment of $48.75

DATE	PATIENT NAME	TREATMENT	CHARGE	PAYMENT	CURRENT BALANCE

16. Use the ledger card to record the following respiratory therapy charges and payments for Jim Bosley. He has a current balance of $379.24.

3/15/–	Initial consultation fee: $125.50
	Chest X rays: 3 at $55.80 each
	Respiratory function tests: 6 at $51.35 each
	Arterial blood gas test: $146.55

Postural drainage treatment: 15 minutes at $94.80 per hour
Payment of $25.00

3/21/–   IPPB (intermittent positive pressure breathing) treatment: 30 minutes at $84.60 per hour
CT (computerized tomography) of lungs: $735.80
Payment of $174.75

3/28/–   Postural drainage treatment: ½ hour
IPPB: 15-minute treatment
Oxygen treatment: ¼ hour at $46.00 per hour
No payment made

3/30/–   Insurance payment ROA (received on account): $571.36

4/04/–   Postural drainage treatment: 45 minutes
IPPB: 30-minute treatment
Oxygen: 15-minute treatment
Payment of $32.75

4/12/–   Respiratory function tests: 2 at $51.35 each
Postural drainage treatment: 20 minutes
IPPB: 20-minute treatment
Payment of $55.75

DATE	PATIENT NAME	TREATMENT	CHARGE	PAYMENT	CURRENT BALANCE

Unit 42 CHECKS, DEPOSIT SLIPS, AND RECEIPTS

BASIC PRINCIPLES FOR WRITING CHECKS, DEPOSIT SLIPS, AND RECEIPTS

Checks:

Checks, deposit slips, and receipts must be completed correctly because they provide a record of financial transactions. A *check* is a written order for payment of money through a bank. Certain terms are associated with checks. A *payee* is the person who receives payment. The *originator* or *maker* is the person writing the check or issuing payment. An *endorsement* is the signature of the payee, usually required on the back of the check before it can be cashed.

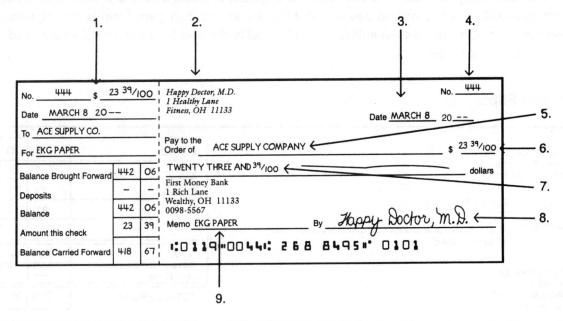

The parts of a check are shown on the sample. They are as follows:

1. The stub or register
2. The name and address of originator or maker
3. The date the check is written
4. The number of the check
5. The payee
6. Amount of check written in numbers

7. Amount of check written in words
8. Signature of originator or maker
9. Memo area for writing reason for check

Checks must always be written in ink to avoid alterations. All notations should be as close to the left side of the line as possible. Cents are usually written as a fraction of one dollar: "—/100."

Before writing a check, it is best to complete the stub or register first by filling in the date, number of check, payee, and reason for the check. The *"Balance Brought Forward"* represents the current balance in the checking account. If any deposits are made to the account they are added to this amount in the areas shown. The amount of the check being written is then subtracted from the current balance in the checkbook to determine the remaining balance. This prevents writing a check without sufficient funds in the account. The final balance is then carried forward to the next check stub or register so it is available when the next check is written. When the stub or register is complete, the check should be written clearly and legibly. Fill in the date, payee, amount of check in numbers, amount of check in words, and a brief memo or reason why the check is written. Only the originator or maker should sign the check. In many health care facilities, an authorized person writes the checks and then gives them to the originator or maker for the proper signature. All entries should be double-checked for accuracy before the check is given or sent to the payee.

Deposit Slips:

Happy Doctor, M.D. 1 Healthy Lane Fitness, OH 11133 Date _____ March 8 _____ 20 — Signature _____ (If cash received) First Money Bank 1 Rich Lane Wealthy, OH 11133 0098-5567	Currency	21	00
	Coin	2	38
	Checks	24	50
		182	06
	TOTAL	229	94
	Less Cash	—	—
	TOTAL DEPOSIT	229	94

A *deposit slip* is a record of money that is deposited in a bank or financial institution. Coins and currency are counted and listed in their correct columns. Checks are usually listed separately on a series of lines. Many deposit slips have room on the back to record a list of checks. They are added together and this total amount is then transferred to the correct area on the front of the deposit slip. If any cash is withheld, a signature of the originator or maker of the account is required on the deposit slip. The total amount deposited must then be added to the next stub or receipt in the checkbook, so the current balance in the checkbook will be accurate.

No. _____	$ _____		
Date_____			
To _____			
For _____			
Balance Brought Forward		418	67
Deposits		229	94
Balance		648	61
Amount this check			
Balance Carried Forward			

The sample shows the stub or register of the next check. The balance brought forward from the previous check is added to the deposit to show the total amount in the checking account.

Receipts:

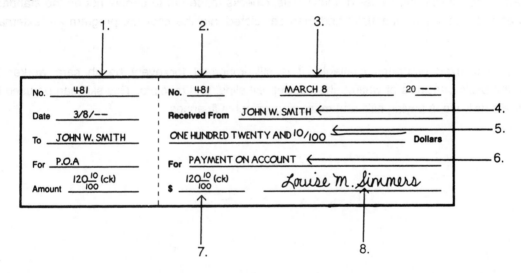

A *receipt* is a record of money or goods received. If a person makes a payment, a receipt can be given to the person as proof of payment. The sample receipt shows the main parts. They are as follows:

1. Stub or register for record
2. Number of receipt
3. Date receipt is written
4. Name of person from whom money was received
5. Amount of money received in words
6. Memo showing reason for payment

7. Amount of money received in numbers with method of payment (check or cash)
8. Signature of person who accepted the payment

Receipts should also be written in ink to avoid alterations. All names and amounts should be written close to the left side of the line. All entries should be double-checked for accuracy before the receipt is given to the patient.

Computerized Checks, Deposit Slips, and Receipts:

Some health care agencies use computer programs to maintain all financial records. Most of the programs will also print checks, deposit slips, and receipts. The software for the programs is user-friendly and easy to use. However, strict controls must be in place to limit access to these programs. Most agencies used password protection to limit the number of individuals who can use the program. In addition, safeguards are added to the programs to prevent an individual from generating a check without documentation in the program for the reason for the check. Some health care agencies restrict the names of payees to standard sources such as utility companies, insurance companies, specific suppliers, and other similar companies or individuals. Checks made out to people not on the standard list of payees must be written manually and then calculated into the financial program as "external" checks.

Even with computerized programs available, it is still important for every health care worker to understand the basic principles of writing checks, deposit slips, and receipts. This skill can be used in any individual's daily life in paying bills and managing personal finances.

PRACTICAL PROBLEMS

1. Write a check for $232.68 to the Illuminating Company for the March electric bill. The balance brought forward in the checking account is $1,014.34.

```
No. ____ $ _____    | Happy Doctor, MD            No. _____
Date _____ 20__    | 1 Healthy Lane
To _____      | Fitness, OH  11133      _____ 20__
For _____       |
                      | Pay to the
_____    | Order of: _____ $___
Balance       |   |   |
Am't Dep.     |   |   | _____ Dollars
Total         |   |   | First Money Bank
Am't Ck.      |   |   | 1 Rich Lane
Balance       |   |   | Wealthy, OH  11133
                      | 00098-5567        By _____
                      | Memo _____
```

2. Write a check for $576.95 to Asco Dental Repair Company for work done on the dental operatory. The balance brought forward in the checking account is $18,017.35.

```
No. ____ $ _____    | Happy Doctor, MD            No. _____
Date _____ 20__    | 1 Healthy Lane
To _____      | Fitness, OH  11133      _____ 20__
For _____       |
                      | Pay to the
_____    | Order of: _____ $___
Balance       |   |   |
Am't Dep.     |   |   | _____ Dollars
Total         |   |   | First Money Bank
Am't Ck.      |   |   | 1 Rich Lane
Balance       |   |   | Wealthy, OH  11133
                      | 00098-5567        By _____
                      | Memo _____
```

3. Complete a deposit slip for the following amounts:

      Coins: $52.73
      Currency: $648.00
      Checks: $76.42, $321.68, and $159.20

Happy Doctor, MD 1 Healthy Lane Fitness, OH 11133 Date _____ 20 ____ Signature _____ (If cash received) First Money Bank 1 Rich Lane Wealthy, OH 11133 0098-5567	Currency		
	Coin		
	Checks ____		
	____		
	____		
	TOTAL		
	Less Cash		
	TOTAL DEPOSIT		

4. Complete a deposit slip with the following amounts calculated:

      Coins: 23 pennies, 27 nickels, 21 dimes, and 42 quarters
      Currency: 56 $1 bills, 33 $5 bills, 27 $10 bills, 16 $20 bills and 5 $50 bills
      Checks: $123.50, $78.65, and $1,211.14

Happy Doctor, MD 1 Healthy Lane Fitness, OH 11133 Date _____ 20 ____ Signature _____ (If cash received) First Money Bank 1 Rich Lane Wealthy, OH 11133 0098-5567	Currency		
	Coin		
	Checks ____		
	____		
	TOTAL		
	Less Cash		
	TOTAL DEPOSIT		

5. Write a receipt to James Johnson for the $156.90 check he paid for his physical examination.

No. _____	No. _____ 20 ___
Date _____	Received From _____
To _____	_____ Dollars
For _____	For _____
Amount _____	$ _____ _____

6. Write a receipt to Virginia Clay for her $78.45 payment in cash for her office visit and medications.

No. _____	No. _____ 20 ___
Date _____	Received From _____
To _____	_____ Dollars
For _____	For _____
Amount _____	$ _____ _____

7. The checking account has a current balance of $1,076.50. Complete the following transactions and balance the account.

a. Write a check for $227.43 to Madison Pharmaceutical for medications.

b. Write a check for $678.53 to Sandusky Medical Equipment for a hemoglobinometer.

c. Write a receipt to Nancy Webber for the $56.75 cash payment she makes for an office visit and blood tests.

d. Write a receipt to Jay Chang for the $226.75 check payment he makes for a physical exam and electrocardigram (ECG).

e. Deposit both Nancy Webber's and Jay Chang's payments into the account by completing a deposit slip.

f. Calculate the current balance in the account by adding the deposit to the stub or register of the next check.

No. ____ $ _____ | Happy Doctor, MD   No. _____
Date _____ 20__ | 1 Healthy Lane
To _____ | Fitness, OH 11133   _____ 20___
For _____ |
                   | Pay to the
_____ | Order of: _____ $____
Balance |
Am't Dep. | _____ Dollars
Total |
Am't Ck. | First Money Bank
Balance | 1 Rich Lane
                   | Wealthy, OH 11133
                   | 00098-5567   By _____
                   | Memo _____

No. ____ $ _____ | Happy Doctor, MD   No. _____
Date _____ 20__ | 1 Healthy Lane
To _____ | Fitness, OH 11133   _____ 20___
For _____ |
                   | Pay to the
_____ | Order of: _____ $____
Balance |
Am't Dep. | _____ Dollars
Total |
Am't Ck. | First Money Bank
Balance | 1 Rich Lane
                   | Wealthy, OH 11133
                   | 00098-5567   By _____
                   | Memo _____

No. _____ | No. _____ 20___
Date _____ | Received From _____
To _____ | _____ Dollars
For _____ | For _____
Amount _____ | $ _____   _____

No. _____   No. _____ 20 ____

Date _____   Received From _____

To _____   _____ Dollars

For _____   For _____

Amount _____ $ _____   _____

Happy Doctor, MD
1 Healthy Lane
Fitness, OH 11133

Date _____ 20 _____
Signature _____
          (If cash received)

First Money Bank
1 Rich Lane
Wealthy, OH 11133
0098-5567

Currency		
Coin		
Checks _____		
_____		
TOTAL		
Less Cash		
TOTAL DEPOSIT		

No. _____ $ _____ | Happy Doctor, MD   No. _____
Date _____ 20__ | 1 Healthy Lane
To _____ | Fitness, OH 11133   _____ 20 ___
For _____ |
                    | Pay to the
                    | Order of: _____ $ ___
Balance |
Am't Dep. | _____ Dollars
Total |
Am't Ck. | First Money Bank
Balance | 1 Rich Lane
                    | Wealthy, OH 11133
                    | 00098-5567   By _____
                    | Memo _____

8. The checking account has a current balance of $24,376.82. Complete the following transactions and balance the account.

   a. Write a check for $1,798.64 to Columbus Dental Supply Company for dental materials.

   b. Write a check for $354.78 to Edison Electric Company for the electric bill.

   c. Write a receipt to Juanita Estridge for the $126.75 cash payment she makes for a dental exam and two amalgam restorations.

   d. Write a receipt to Tyronne Trent for the $895.74 check payment he makes for a mandibular denture.

   e. Deposit both Juanita Estridge's and Tyronne Trent's payments into the account by completing a deposit slip.

   f. Calculate the current balance in the account by adding the deposit to the stub or register of the next check.

No. _____ $ _____ | Happy Doctor, MD   No. _____

Date _____ 20__ | 1 Healthy Lane

To _____ | Fitness, OH 11133   _____ 20___

For _____ |

                    | Pay to the

_____ | Order of: _____ $____

Balance | |

Am't Dep. | | _____ Dollars

Total | |

Am't Ck. | | First Money Bank

Balance | | 1 Rich Lane

                    | Wealthy, OH 11133

                    | 00098-5567   By _____

                    | Memo _____

No. _____ | No. _____ 20___

Date _____ | Received From _____

To _____ | _____ Dollars

For _____ | For _____

Amount _____ | $ _____   _____

No. _____ | No. _____ 20___

Date _____ | Received From _____

To _____ | _____ Dollars

For _____ | For _____

Amount _____ | $ _____   _____

Happy Doctor, MD
1 Healthy Lane
Fitness, OH 11133

Date _____ 20 _____
Signature _____
                (If cash received)

First Money Bank
1 Rich Lane
Wealthy, OH 11133
0098-5567

Currency		
Coin		
Checks _____		
_____		
TOTAL		
Less Cash		
TOTAL DEPOSIT		

No. ____ $ _____
Date _____ 20 ___
To _____
For _____

Balance		
Am't Dep.		
Total		
Am't Ck.		
Balance		

Happy Doctor, MD
1 Healthy Lane
Fitness, OH 11133

Pay to the
Order of: _____

First Money Bank
1 Rich Lane
Wealthy, OH 11133
00098-5567
Memo _____

No. _____

_____ 20 ___

_____ $ ____

_____ Dollars

By _____

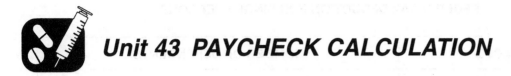 # Unit 43 PAYCHECK CALCULATION

BASIC PRINCIPLES OF PAYCHECK CALCULATION

Every individual should be able to calculate a paycheck. Two main terms are used regarding payroll: gross pay and net pay. *Gross pay* is the total amount of money earned for hours worked. *Net pay*, often called "take-home pay," is the amount of money left after all deductions have been subtracted from the gross pay. Some common deductions are federal income tax, state income tax, city/township tax, and FICA (Social Security).

Calculating Gross Pay:

To determine gross pay, multiply the wage per hour times the number of hours worked. Overtime pay is usually calculated at time and a half or double time. If overtime is one and a half, multiply the overtime hours by 1.5 and then multiply by the wage per hour. For double time, multiply the overtime hours by two and then multiply by the wage per hour.

Example: A geriatric assistant earns $7.45 per hour. If he works 40 hours of regular time and 6 hours of overtime at time and a half, what is his gross pay?

Hourly wage	×	Hours worked			=	Regular Gross Pay
$7.45	×	40			=	$298.00
Hourly wage	×	Hours worked	×	1.5	=	Overtime Gross Pay
$7.45	×	6	×	1.5	=	$67.05
Regular Gross Pay	+	Overtime Gross Pay			=	Total Gross Pay
$298.00	+	$67.05			=	$365.05

Calculating Net Pay:

To determine net pay, individual deductions must be calculated first. The deduction for federal income tax is based on salary earned, marital status, and the number of dependents claimed. A dependent is claimed for each individual supported by the person earning a wage. For example, a woman supporting two children would claim three dependents, one for herself and one for each of the children. Tables are used to determine the appropriate deduction.

It is important to use the most recent tax tables available. Tax laws change frequently. The most recent tax tables can be found at the Internet site for the Internal Revenue Service. Most health care agencies use special software programs that automatically calculate the correct federal tax deduction depending on gross income, marital status, and number of dependents. The software has to be updated at frequent intervals to ensure that the correct amount of federal tax deduction is withheld from a person's gross pay. Two sample federal tax withholding tables are shown, one for single persons and one for married persons.

FEDERAL TAX DEDUCTION FOR SINGLE PERSONS

WAGES		NUMBER OF DEPENDENTS			
AT LEAST	LESS THAN	0	1	2	3
$ 270.00	$ 280.00	$ 26.05	$ 24.39	$ 23.56	$ 22.73
$ 280.00	$ 290.00	$ 27.55	$ 25.69	$ 24.76	$ 23.83
$ 290.00	$ 300.00	$ 29.05	$ 26.99	$ 25.96	$ 24.93
$ 300.00	$ 310.00	$ 30.55	$ 28.29	$ 27.16	$ 26.03
$ 310.00	$ 320.00	$ 32.05	$ 29.59	$ 28.36	$ 27.13
$ 320.00	$ 330.00	$ 33.55	$ 30.89	$ 29.56	$ 28.23
$ 330.00	$ 340.00	$ 35.05	$ 32.19	$ 30.76	$ 29.33
$ 340.00	$ 350.00	$ 36.55	$ 33.49	$ 31.96	$ 30.43
$ 350.00	$ 360.00	$ 38.05	$ 34.79	$ 33.16	$ 31.53
$ 360.00	$ 370.00	$ 39.55	$ 36.09	$ 34.36	$ 32.63
$ 370.00	$ 380.00	$ 41.05	$ 37.39	$ 35.56	$ 33.73
$ 380.00	$ 390.00	$ 42.55	$ 38.69	$ 36.76	$ 34.83
$ 390.00	$ 400.00	$ 44.05	$ 39.99	$ 37.96	$ 35.93
$ 400.00	$ 410.00	$ 45.55	$ 41.29	$ 39.16	$ 37.03
$ 410.00	$ 420.00	$ 47.05	$ 42.59	$ 40.36	$ 38.13
$ 420.00	$ 430.00	$ 48.55	$ 43.89	$ 41.56	$ 39.23
$ 430.00	$ 440.00	$ 50.05	$ 45.19	$ 42.76	$ 40.33
$ 440.00	$ 450.00	$ 51.55	$ 46.49	$ 43.96	$ 41.43
$ 450.00	$ 460.00	$ 53.05	$ 47.79	$ 45.16	$ 42.53
$ 460.00	$ 470.00	$ 54.55	$ 49.09	$ 46.36	$ 43.63
$ 470.00	$ 480.00	$ 56.05	$ 50.39	$ 47.56	$ 44.73
$ 480.00	$ 490.00	$ 57.55	$ 51.69	$ 48.76	$ 45.83
$ 490.00	$ 500.00	$ 59.05	$ 52.99	$ 49.96	$ 46.93
$ 500.00	$ 510.00	$ 60.55	$ 54.29	$ 51.16	$ 48.03
$ 510.00	$ 520.00	$ 62.05	$ 55.59	$ 52.36	$ 49.13
$ 520.00	$ 530.00	$ 63.55	$ 56.89	$ 53.56	$ 50.23
$ 530.00	$ 540.00	$ 65.05	$ 58.19	$ 54.76	$ 51.33
$ 540.00	$ 550.00	$ 66.55	$ 59.49	$ 55.96	$ 52.43
$ 550.00	$ 560.00	$ 68.05	$ 60.79	$ 57.16	$ 53.53

FEDERAL TAX DEDUCTION FOR MARRIED PERSONS

WAGES		NUMBER OF DEPENDENTS			
AT LEAST	LESS THAN	0	1	2	3
$ 270.00	$ 280.00	$ 23.62	$ 22.42	$ 21.24	$ 20.06
$ 280.00	$ 290.00	$ 24.62	$ 23.37	$ 22.14	$ 20.91
$ 290.00	$ 300.00	$ 25.63	$ 24.32	$ 23.04	$ 21.76
$ 300.00	$ 310.00	$ 26.63	$ 25.27	$ 23.94	$ 22.61
$ 310.00	$ 320.00	$ 27.63	$ 26.22	$ 24.84	$ 23.46
$ 320.00	$ 330.00	$ 28.63	$ 27.17	$ 25.74	$ 24.31
$ 330.00	$ 340.00	$ 29.63	$ 28.12	$ 26.64	$ 25.16
$ 340.00	$ 350.00	$ 30.63	$ 29.07	$ 27.54	$ 26.01
$ 350.00	$ 360.00	$ 31.63	$ 30.02	$ 28.44	$ 26.86
$ 360.00	$ 370.00	$ 32.63	$ 30.97	$ 29.34	$ 27.71
$ 370.00	$ 380.00	$ 33.63	$ 31.92	$ 30.24	$ 28.56
$ 380.00	$ 390.00	$ 34.63	$ 32.87	$ 31.14	$ 29.41
$ 390.00	$ 400.00	$ 35.64	$ 33.82	$ 32.04	$ 30.26
$ 400.00	$ 410.00	$ 36.64	$ 34.77	$ 32.94	$ 31.11
$ 410.00	$ 420.00	$ 37.64	$ 35.72	$ 33.84	$ 31.96
$ 420.00	$ 430.00	$ 38.64	$ 36.67	$ 34.74	$ 32.81
$ 430.00	$ 440.00	$ 39.64	$ 37.62	$ 35.64	$ 33.66
$ 440.00	$ 450.00	$ 40.64	$ 38.57	$ 36.54	$ 34.51
$ 450.00	$ 460.00	$ 41.64	$ 39.52	$ 37.44	$ 35.36
$ 460.00	$ 470.00	$ 42.64	$ 40.47	$ 38.34	$ 36.21
$ 470.00	$ 480.00	$ 43.64	$ 41.42	$ 39.24	$ 37.06
$ 480.00	$ 490.00	$ 44.64	$ 42.37	$ 40.14	$ 37.91
$ 490.00	$ 500.00	$ 45.65	$ 43.32	$ 41.04	$ 38.76
$ 500.00	$ 510.00	$ 46.65	$ 44.27	$ 41.94	$ 39.61
$ 510.00	$ 520.00	$ 47.65	$ 45.22	$ 42.84	$ 40.46
$ 520.00	$ 530.00	$ 48.65	$ 46.17	$ 43.74	$ 41.31
$ 530.00	$ 540.00	$ 49.65	$ 47.12	$ 44.64	$ 42.16
$ 540.00	$ 550.00	$ 50.65	$ 48.07	$ 45.54	$ 43.01
$ 550.00	$ 560.00	$ 51.65	$ 49.02	$ 46.44	$ 43.86

To use one of the tables, first find the table with the appropriate marital status, either married or single. Then use the left columns to locate the gross pay earned. Find the column with the correct number of dependents and use the amount shown as the deduction for federal tax.

Example: A geriatric assistant earns $365.05 total gross pay in one week. He is married and claims 3 dependents. What amount should be deducted for federal income tax?

Use the "Federal Tax Deduction for Married Persons" table.

Find the salary listing between $360 and $370.

Trace over to the column showing 3 dependents.

The amount to deduct for federal income tax is $27.71.

To calculate the deduction for state income tax, similar tables are available in many states. In other states, the state income tax is a percent of gross income. The deduction is determined by multiplying the state percent times the gross pay.

Example: A geriatric assistant earns a gross pay of $365.05 for one week. His state income tax is $2\frac{1}{2}$ percent, or 0.025 when converted to decimals. What is the deduction for state income tax?

Gross Pay $\times$ Percent of Tax = Deduction for State Tax
$365.05 $\times$ 0.025 ($2\frac{1}{2}$%) = $9.12625
$9.13 = Deduction for State Tax

City or township taxes are usually a percent of gross income and are calculated the same way state tax is calculated. The gross income is multiplied by the percent of the tax to obtain the proper deduction.

Example: A geriatric assistant earns a gross pay of $365.05 for one week. His city income tax is $1\frac{1}{4}$ percent, or 0.0125 when converted to decimals. What is the deduction for city income tax?

Gross Pay $\times$ Percent of Tax = Deduction for City Tax
$365.05 $\times$ 0.0125 ($1\frac{1}{4}$%) = $4.563125
$4.56 = Deduction for City Tax

The deduction for FICA (Social Security) includes 6.2% of the first $87,200 income and a Medicare deduction of 1.45% of the total in income for a total deduction of 7.65%, or 0.0765 in decimals. The gross pay is multiplied by this percent to obtain the correct deduction for FICA.

Example: A geriatric assistant earns a gross pay of $365.05 per week. What is the deduction for FICA?

Gross Pay $\times$ FICA Percent = Deduction for FICA
$365.05 $\times$ 0.0765 (7.65%) = $27.926325
27.93 = Deduction for FICA

To calculate the net pay, all of the deductions must be subtracted from the gross pay. Many health care facilities use computer programs or special cards to record these calculations.

TIME AND SALARY COMPUTATION RECORD

Name _Greene, Mike_   SS _000-11-5111_   Date _10/11/– to 10/17/–_
Marital Status _M_   Dependents _3_   Pay Rate _$7.45_

DATES	ON	OFF	HOURS	PAY CALCULATION	AMOUNTS	
10/11/–	7 AM	3 PM	8	Regular Pay: 40 x 7.45	298	00
10/12/–	7 AM	3 PM	8	Overtime Pay: 6 x 1.5 x 7.45	67	05
10/13/–	7 AM	3 PM	8	**TOTAL GROSS WAGES**	365	05
10/14/–				Deductions:		
10/15/–	7 AM	3 PM	8	Federal Withholding Tax	27	71
10/16/–	7 AM	3 PM	8	State Tax	9	13
10/17/–	7 AM	1 PM	6	City Tax	4	56
				FICA	27	93
				Other:		
				TOTAL DEDUCTIONS	69	33
TOTALS	**BASE: 40**	**OT: 6**		**AMOUNT OF CHECK**	295	72

The sample time and salary card shows the dates and hours worked. The gross pay is calculated from regular pay and overtime pay. The deductions are itemized in the right-hand column under deductions. All of the deductions are added together and then subtracted from the gross pay to obtain the net pay of $295.72, shown as "Amount of Check" on the card.

PRACTICAL PROBLEMS

1. A veterinary technician (VTR) works 36 hours at an hourly wage of $8.48. What is his gross pay?   _____

2. A physical therapist (PT) works 40 hours of regular time and 7 hours of overtime at double time. Her hourly wage is $16.20. What is her gross pay?   _____

3. A registered nurse (RN) works 47½ hours at an hourly wage of $18.72. He earns time and a half for all hours over 40 hours. What is his gross pay?   _____

4. A pharmacy technician works 7 hours per day for 4 days and 8 hours per day for 2 days. She earns $8.19 per hour and gets time and a half for all hours over 40 hours. What is her gross pay?   _____

5. Use the federal tax deduction tables to determine the federal income tax deduction for the following individuals.

   a. An occupational therapist (OT) earns $492.76 gross pay. She is married and claims 2 dependents.   _____

   b. An electrocardiograph (ECG) technician earns $312.87 gross pay. He is single and claims 1 dependent.   _____

   c. A dental hygienist (DH) earns $534.38 gross pay. He is single and claims 2 dependents.   _____

   d. A medical lab technician (MLT) earns $489.08 gross pay. She is married and claims 3 dependents.   _____

6. A dental assistant (DA) earns $342.95 gross pay. She is married and claims 2 dependents. Her state tax is 3%, city tax is 1%, and FICA is 7.65%. What is her net pay? (*Hint:* Remember to multiply all percents times the gross pay to determine all deductions.)   _____

7. A licensed practical nurse (LPN) working part-time earns $394.28 gross pay. He is single and claims 1 dependent. State tax is 4%, city tax is $1\frac{1}{2}$%, and FICA is 7.65%. What is his net pay?   _____

8. A medical secretary earns $274.59 gross pay. She is single and claims 2 dependents. State tax is $3\frac{1}{2}$%, city tax is 2%, and FICA is 7.65%. What is her net pay?   _____

9. An ambulance dispatcher earns $7.94 per hour. He works 37 hours in one week. He is single and claims 1 dependent. State tax is $3\frac{1}{2}$%, city tax is $1\frac{1}{2}$%, and FICA is 7.65%. What is his net pay?   _____

10. A public health educator earns $14.10 per hour. She works 28 hours. She is married and claims 3 dependents. State tax is $2\frac{1}{4}$%, city tax is $1\frac{1}{4}$%, and FICA is 7.65%. What is her net pay?   _____

11. A part-time clinic nurse earns a yearly gross salary of $18,564. He is paid every week. He is married and claims 2 dependents. State tax is 2%, township tax is $1\frac{1}{2}$%, and FICA is 7.65%. What is his weekly net income? (*Hint:* To determine gross pay per week, divide the yearly salary by the number of weeks per year.)   _____

12. An adolescent counselor earns $27,216 gross pay per year and is paid weekly. She is single and claims 2 dependents. State tax is 4%, city tax is $1\frac{3}{4}$%, and FICA is 7.65%. What is her weekly net pay?   _____

13. An admissions clerk at a hospital earns $7.12 per hour. One week he works 40 hours of regular time and 5 hours of overtime at double time. He is single and claims 0 dependents. State tax is $4\frac{1}{4}$%, city tax is $2\frac{1}{2}$%, and FICA is 7.65%. What is his net pay?

_____

14. A radiologic assistant earns double time for all hours over 8 hours per day. She works 4 days for 10 hours per day and earns $8.23 per hour. She is married and claims 2 dependents. State tax is $3\frac{3}{4}$%, city tax is $2\frac{1}{2}$%, and FICA is 7.65%. What is her net pay?

_____

15. A certified ophthalmalic technician (COT) earns time and a half for all hours over 40 per week. However, he also earns double time for any hours over 8 hours per day. One week he works 2 days for 10 hours, 3 days for 8 hours, and one day for 4 hours. He earns $10.18 per hour. He is married and claims 3 dependents. State tax is $3\frac{3}{4}$%, city tax is $1\frac{1}{4}$%, and FICA is 7.65%. What is his net pay for the week?

_____

16. Complete the time and salary record showing the total hours worked, total earnings, individual deductions, total deductions, and amount of check. The person is single and claims 1 dependent. All hours over 40 are calculated at the overtime rate.

TIME AND SALARY COMPUTATION RECORD

Name _____ SS _____ Date _____

Marital Status *S* Dependents *1* Pay Rate *$8.55*

DATES	ON	OFF	HOURS	PAY CALCULATION	AMOUNTS	
11/03/–				Regular Pay:		
11/04/–	6 AM	2 PM	8	Overtime Pay: 1.5 x		
11/05/–	8 AM	4 PM	8	**TOTAL GROSS WAGES**		
11/06/–	6 AM	4 PM	10	Deductions:		
11/07/–				Federal Withholding Tax		
11/08/–	7 AM	5 PM	10	State Tax: 5%		
11/09/–				City Tax: 1.5%		
				FICA: 7.65%		
				Other:		
				TOTAL DEDUCTIONS		
TOTALS	**BASE:**	**OT:**		**AMOUNT OF CHECK**		

17. Complete the time and salary record showing the total hours worked, total earnings, individual deductions, total deductions, and amount of check. All hours over 40 hours are calculated at the overtime rate. The person is married and claims 2 dependents.

TIME AND SALARY COMPUTATION RECORD

Name _____   SS _____   Date _____

Marital Status __M____   Dependents __2____   Pay Rate ___$9.13_____

DATES	ON	OFF	HOURS	PAY CALCULATION	AMOUNTS	
12/08/–	6 AM	3 PM		Regular Pay:		
12/09/–	6 AM	3 PM		Overtime Pay: 1.5 x		
12/10/–	8 AM	6 PM		**TOTAL GROSS WAGES**		
12/11/–				Deductions:		
12/12/–	7 AM	3 PM		Federal Withholding Tax		
12/13/–	6 AM	3 PM		State Tax: 3%		
12/14/–	7 AM	11 AM		City Tax: 2.5%		
				FICA: 7.65%		
				Other:		
				TOTAL DEDUCTIONS		
TOTALS	**BASE:**	**OT:**		**AMOUNT OF CHECK**		

18. Complete the time and salary record showing the total hours worked, total earnings, individual deductions, total deductions, and amount of check. Any hours over 8 hours per day are calculated at double time. Any hours over 40 hours per week are calculated at time and a half. The person is single and claims 1 dependent.

TIME AND SALARY COMPUTATION RECORD

Name _____   SS _____   Date _____

Marital Status __S__   Dependents __1__   Pay Rate __$7.94__

DATES	ON	OFF	HOURS	PAY CALCULATION	AMOUNTS	
01/05/–	2 PM	11 PM	9	Regular Pay:		
01/06/–	3 PM	8 PM	5	Overtime Pay:		
01/07/–	2 PM	11 PM	9	**TOTAL GROSS WAGES**		
01/08/–	2 PM	10 PM	8	Deductions:		
01/09/–				Federal Withholding Tax		
01/10/–	1 PM	10 PM	9	State Tax: 4⅖%		
01/11/–	5 PM	10 PM	5	City Tax: 1⅛%		
				FICA: 7.65%		
				Other:		
				TOTAL DEDUCTIONS		
TOTALS	**BASE:**	**OT:**		**AMOUNT OF CHECK**		

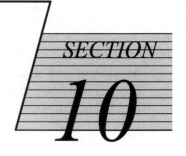

Math for Medications

Unit 44 CALCULATING ORAL DOSAGE

BASIC PRINCIPLES OF CALCULATING ORAL DOSAGE

An oral medication is a medication taken by mouth. It is the most common route for administration of medications. Oral medications are available in solid forms such as tablets, capsules, powders, and lozenges, or in liquid forms such as solutions, elixirs, suspensions, and syrups.

Proportional Method of Calculating Oral Dosage:

Two main methods are used to calculate oral dosage: the proportional method and the formula method. To use the proportional method, all units of measurement must be the same. For example, if the ordered medication is in grams and the medication is available in milligrams, the units must be converted to the same unit of measurement, either grams or milligrams. If necessary, review Section 6 to perform the conversions. Once the units of measurement are the same, a proportion is created to represent the information.

Example: A doctor orders 300 milligrams (mg) of Floxin®, an antibiotic. Capsules available contain 100 mg per capsule.

$$\frac{\text{Known dosage available}}{\text{Known dosage form}} = \frac{\text{Dosage ordered}}{\text{Amount to be given}}$$

$$\frac{100 \text{ mg}}{1 \text{ capsule}} \qquad \underset{=}{\times} \qquad \frac{300 \text{ mg}}{X \text{ capsules}} \quad (X \text{ is unknown.})$$

Product of means equals product of extremes (Review Unit 21.)

100 mg $\times$ X capsules $=$ 1 capsule $\times$ 300 mg

$100X = 300$ (Divide both sides by 100 to get X alone.)

$100X/100 = 300/100$

$X = 3$ The answer is 3 capsules for the correct dosage.

Formula Method of Calculating Oral Dosage:

To use the formula method, all units of measurement must be the same. Numbers are then inserted into the formula to find the correct amount of medication.

Example: A doctor orders 300 milligrams (mg) of Floxin®, an antibiotic. Capsules available contain 100 mg per capsule.

$$\frac{\text{Dosage ordered}}{\text{Dosage available}} \quad \times \quad \text{Known dosage form} \quad = \quad \text{Amount to give}$$

$$\frac{300 \text{ mg}}{100 \text{ mg}} \quad \times \quad 1 \text{ capsule} \quad = \quad X \text{ capsules } (X \text{ is unknown.})$$

$3 \times 1 = 3$ The answer is 3 capsules for correct dosage.

Calculating Oral Liquid Dosages:

To calculate oral liquid amounts, the same procedures are used, but the liquid amount is used in place of the capsule.

Example: A doctor orders 300 milligrams (mg) of terramycin suspension, an antibiotic. The dosage available contains 0.1 gm per 5 milliliters (ml).

In this case one dosage is in milligrams and the second dosage is in grams. All units of measurement must be the same. The 0.1 grams (gm) must be converted to milligrams (mg).

Known fact: 1 gm = 1000 mg

Set up a proportion

$$\frac{1 \text{ gm}}{1000 \text{ mg}} \quad = \quad \frac{0.1 \text{ gm}}{X \text{ mg}}$$

$1 \times X \qquad = \qquad 0.1 \times 1000$

$1X = 100$

$X = 100$ mg

Now the problem can be solved using 100 mg in place of the 0.1 gm.

Proportional Method:

$$\frac{\text{Known dosage available}}{\text{Known dosage form}} = \frac{\text{Dosage ordered}}{\text{Amount to be given}}$$

$$\frac{100 \text{ mg}}{5 \text{ ml}} \quad\underset{=}{\times}\quad \frac{300 \text{ mg}}{X \text{ ml}} \qquad (X \text{ is unknown.})$$

$100 \text{ mg} \times X \text{ ml} = 5 \text{ ml} \times 300 \text{ mg}$

$100X = 1500$ (Divide both sides by 100 to get X alone.)

$100X/100 = 1500/100$

$X = 15$ The correct dosage is 15 ml.

Formula Method:

$$\frac{\text{Dosage ordered}}{\text{Dosage available}} \times \text{Known dosage form} = \text{Amount to give}$$

$$\frac{300 \text{ mg}}{100 \text{ mg}} \times 5 \text{ ml} = X \text{ ml} \ (X \text{ is unknown.})$$

$3 \times 5 = 15$ The answer is 15 ml for correct dosage.

PRACTICAL PROBLEMS

1. A physician orders 600 milligrams (mg) of potassium chloride (KCl) for a patient taking diuretics. Tablets available contain 300 mg per tablet. How many tablets should be given?   _____

2. A physician orders 500 mg of amoxicillin for a patient with an ear infection. Capsules available contain 250 mg per capsule. How many capsules should be given?   _____

3. A physician orders 250 mg of sulfasalazine for a patient with rheumatoid arthritis. Tablets available contain 500 mg per tablet. How many tablets should be given?   _____

4. A physician orders gr ½ of phenobarbital tablets. How many tablets should be given?   _____

XV 0280 AMX

PHENOBARBITAL
TABLETS, U. S. P.

15 mg (gr 1/4)

Warning: May be habit forming

5. A physician orders 15 mg of prednisone for a patient with an inflammatory joint disease. Tablets available contain 5 mg per tablet. How many tablets should be given?   _____

6. A physician orders 50 mg of Vistaril® suspension to stop the itching for a patient with severe poison ivy. It is available as 25 mg per 5 milliliters (ml). How many ml should be given?   _____

7. A physician orders 50,000 units of Nilstat® suspension for a patient with a skin infection. How many ml should be given?   _____

60 Milliliters

NILSTAT® SUSPENSION
Nystatin, U.S.P

100,000 units in 2 milliliters

8. A physician orders gr (grain) ¼ of morphine for a patient with severe pain from bone cancer. It is available in gr ½ tablets. How many tablets should be given?   _____

9. A physician orders gr X of aspirin for a patient with a high fever. It is available in gr V tablets. How many tablets should be given? (*Hint:* Review Unit 26 on Roman numerals.)   _____

10. A physician orders 0.125 mg of digoxin for a patient with congestive heart failure. How many tablets should be given?   _____

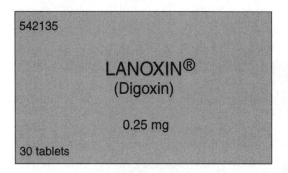

542135

LANOXIN®
(Digoxin)

0.25 mg

30 tablets

11. A physician orders 10 mg of Nembutal® elixir to treat a patient with insomnia. It is available as 20 mg in 5 ml. How many ml should be given?   _____

12. A physician orders 1 gram (gm) of Keflex® for a patient with a streptococcus infection. How many capsules should be given? (*Hint:* All units of measurement must be the same. Review Unit 23 on mass or weight measurements.)   _____

100 Capsules

KEFLEX® CAPSULES
Cephalexin, U.S.P

250 mg

13. A physician orders 0.1 gram (gm) of meprobamate for a patient with anxiety. It is available in 200-milligram (mg) tablets. How many tablets should be given?   _____

14. A physician orders 20 mg of simethicone for a patient with indigestion. It is available as 0.04 gm per 0.6 ml. How many ml should be given?   _____

15. A physician orders 60 mEq (milliequivalents) of potassium gluconate elixir for a patient with hypokalemia (low levels of potassium in the blood) caused by diabetic acidosis. How many teaspoons should be given? (*Hint:* 1 tsp = 5 ml.)   _____

LP-53000-2

POTASSIUM GLUCONATE ELIXIR

20 mEq/15 cc

100 cc

16. A physician orders 0.25 mg of Levsin® drops to treat a patient with irritable bowel syndrome. It is available as 0.125 mg per ml. How many drops should be given? (*Hint:* Review Unit 24 on volume or liquid measurements.)   _____

17. A physician orders gr $\frac{1}{300}$ of atropine to be given to a patient preoperatively (before surgery) to decrease salivary and bronchial secretions. It is available in gr $\frac{1}{150}$ tablets. How many tablets should be given?   _____

18. A physician orders gr $4\frac{1}{2}$ of secobarbital sodium to be taken at HS (bedtime) to induce sleep. How many capsules should be given?   _____

50 Capsules

SECONAL® SODIUM
Secobarbital Sodium, U.S.P

100 mg (grs $1\frac{1}{2}$)

19. A physician orders 8 ml of codeine phosphate syrup for a patient with a severe cough. It is available in gr $\frac{1}{6}$ per 4 ml. How many grains does the patient receive?   _____

20. A physician orders 5 ml of phenobarbital elixir for a patient with seizures caused by meningitis. It is available as 0.03 gm per 7.5 ml. How many mg does the patient receive?   _____

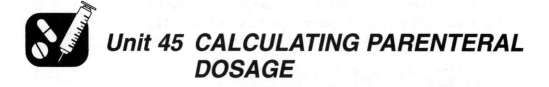

Unit 45 CALCULATING PARENTERAL DOSAGE

BASIC PRINCIPLES OF CALCULATING PARENTERAL DOSAGE

Parenteral medications are medications that are injected into the body. Some different types of injections include subcutaneous (SC) injected just below the surface of the skin, intramuscular (IM) injected into a muscle, and intravenous (IV) injected into a vein. Parenteral medications are supplied as liquids since they are injected into the body. The strength of the medication is usually written as a measurement of weight (milligrams, grams, grains, units) in a measurement of volume (milliliters, cubic centimeters, minims), such as 250 mg/ml. Syringes are used to measure the proper volume amount that is given. Correct dosage for parenteral medications can be calculated by using either the proportion method or the formula method used to calculate oral dosage. It is important to remember that all units of measurement must be the same.

Example: A doctor orders streptomycin 500 mg IM. The dosage available for use contains 1 gram per 2 milliliters. How many ml should be injected?

All units must be in the same unit of measurement.

Convert 1 gram (gm) to milligrams (mg). (Review Unit 23.)

1 gm = 1000 mg

Proportional Method:

$$\frac{\text{Known dosage available}}{\text{Known dosage form}} \quad = \quad \frac{\text{Dosage ordered}}{\text{Amount to be given}}$$

$$\frac{1000 \text{ mg}}{2 \text{ ml}} \quad \bowtie \quad \frac{500 \text{ mg}}{X \text{ ml}} \qquad (X \text{ is unknown.})$$

1000 mg $\times$ X ml = 2 ml $\times$ 500 mg

1000X = 1000   (Divide both sides by 1000 to get X alone.)

1000X/1000 = 1000/1000

X =1   The correct dosage is 1 ml.

Formula Method:

$$\frac{\text{Dosage ordered}}{\text{Dosage available}} \times \text{Known dosage form} = \text{Amount to give}$$

$$\frac{500 \text{ mg}}{1000 \text{ mg}} \times 2 \text{ ml} = X \text{ ml} \ (X \text{ is unknown.})$$

$$\frac{500}{1000} \times 2 = X$$

$\frac{1}{2} \times 2 = 1$ The correct dosage is 1 ml.

PRACTICAL PROBLEMS

1. The physician orders 75 milligrams (mg) of Demerol® IM q4h (every four hours) prn (whenever necessary) for pain. It is available as 50 mg per milliliters (ml). How many ml should be injected?   _____

2. The physician orders Librium® 50 mg IM to relax a patient suffering from alcohol withdrawal. It is available as 100 mg per 2 ml. How many ml should be injected?   _____

3. A physician orders 25 mg of Dilantin® IV for an epileptic with severe psychomotor seizures. It is available as 50 mg per ml. How many ml should be injected?   _____

4. A physician orders 250 mg of Pronestyl® IM for a patient with a ventricular arrhythmia (abnormal heart rhythm). How many ml should be injected?   _____

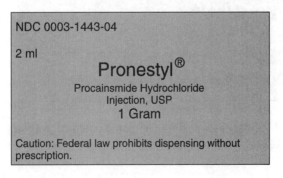

NDC 0003-1443-04

2 ml

Pronestyl®
Procainsmide Hydrochloride
Injection, USP
1 Gram

Caution: Federal law prohibits dispensing without prescription.

5. A physician orders 20 mEq (milliequivalents) of potassium chloride (KCl) IV for a patient with hypokalemia. It is available as 40 mEq per 20 ml. How many ml should be injected?   _____

6. A physician orders 1000 mg of Amikin® IM for a patient with a postop (after surgery) infection. How many ml should be injected?   _____

> **NDC 0015-3020-20**
>
> ## *AMIKIN®*
> *Amikacin Sulfate Injection*
> *For IM or IV Use*
>
> **500 mg per 2 ml**

7. A physician orders 250 mg of Pollycillin-N® IM for a patient with an infected foot. It is available in 1000 mg per 5 ml. How many ml should be injected?   _____

8. A physician orders 100,000 units (U) of Penicillin IM for a patient with syphilis. It is available as 5,000,000 U per 25 ml. How many ml should be injected?   _____

9. A physician orders an injection of 45 micrograms (mcg) of Vitamin B_{12} for a patient with pernicious anemia. It is available as 300 mcg in 10 ml. How many ml should be injected?   _____

10. A physician orders 10 mg of Valium® IM to relax a psychotic patient. How many ml should be injected?   _____

> **10 ml Multiple Dose Vial**
>
> ## *VALIUM®*
> *Diazepam/Roche Injection*
> *For IM or IV Use*
>
> **5 mg per ml**

11. A physician orders 60 mg of gentamicin sulfate IM for a patient with a staphylococcus urinary tract infection. It is available as 80 mg per 2 ml. How many ml should be injected?   _____

12. A physician orders 0.1 mg of atropine IM for a patient with bronchial spasms. It is available as 0.4 mg per ml. How many ml should be injected?   _____

13. A physician orders 2000 mg of Tazicef® IV q12h for a patient with pneumonia. Tazicef® must be reconstituted before use. This means a specific amount of sterile or bacteriostatic water for injection must be added to the powder in the vial to create a solution of Tazicef®. Read the label carefully.

NDC 0007-5086-01 Equivalent to *6 Grams* of ceftazidime *TAZICEF®* Ceftazidime for Injection Pharmacy Bulk Vial Federal Law prohibits dispensing without a prescription.	**Before reconstitution:** Protect from light and store at controlled temperature (59° to 96°F). **Reconstitution:** Add Sterile water or Bacteriostatic water for injection according to amounts below. SHAKE WELL before using. Concentration Amount of Dilutent 1 gm/5 ml 26 ml 1 gm/10 ml 56 ml

a. If the Tazicef® is reconstituted with 26 ml of dilutent, how many ml would have to be given to the patient? _____

b. If the Tazicef® is reconstituted with 56 ml of dilutent, how many ml would have to be given to the patient? _____

14. A physician orders 250 mg of Keflin® IM for a patient with an infection. It is available as 1 gram (gm) per 10 ml. How many ml should be injected? (*Hint:* Remember that all units of measurement must be the same.) _____

15. A patient is given 1.5 ml of Kefsol® IM.

NDC 0002-1497-01 ***KEFSOL®*** *Sterile Cefazolin Sodium* *For IM or IV Use* **1 gm per 2 ml**

a. How many grams of Kefsol® are injected? _____

b. How many mg of Kefsol® are injected? _____

16. A patient is given 15 ml of Isuprel® in an IV drip. It is available as 1 mg in 5 ml. How many mg are injected?

_____

17. A patient is given 2 ml of Dilaudid® IM. It is available as 50 mg per 5 ml. How many mg are injected?

_____

18. A physician orders an IV drip containing 400,000 units of penicillin G for a patient with otitis media (middle ear infection). Read the following label carefully.

NDC 0003-0668-05 5,000,000 units per vial **PENICILLIN G SODIUM** for INJECTION USP	**Sterile: For intramuscular or intravenous drip use** Store at room temperature prior to constitution.
	Preparation of Solution: Add 23 ml, 18 ml, 8 ml, or 3 ml sterile water for injection diluent to provide 200,000 *u*, 250,000 *u*, 500,000 *u*, or 1,000,000 *u* per ml respectively.
Federal Law prohibits dispensing without a prescription.	Sterile solution may be kept in refrigerator 1 week without significant loss of potency.

a. If 23 ml of dilutent is used to reconstitute the penicillin G, how many ml should be injected?

_____

b. If 8 ml of dilutent is used to reconstitute the penicillin G, how many ml should be injected?

_____

c. If 3 ml of dilutent is used to reconstitute the penicillin G, how many ml should be injected?

_____

19. A physician orders 200 mg of acyclovir IV for a patient with shingles. Acyclovir comes in a powdered form in a 0.5-gm vial. The directions state it should be reconstituted with 5 ml of normal saline. How many ml would contain the ordered dosage?

_____

20. Heparin is an anticoagulant that is used to prevent the blood from clotting. It is measured in USP units. The major routes of administration are IV or deep subcutaneous. It is not effective if given orally and is never given intramuscularly. Extreme care must be used to administer the exact dosage prescribed. A tuberculin syringe (review Unit 32) is usually used. Heparin is available in a wide variety of strengths to reduce dosage errors. Strengths available include 1000 units per ml, 2500 units per ml, 5000 units per ml, 7500 units per ml, 10,000 units per ml, and 20,000 units per ml. Read the labels carefully.

NDC 0009-0268-02
30 ml

Heparin Sodium
Injection, USP

Sterile Solution from beef lung

1,000 Units per ml

For subcutaneous or intravenous use

NDC 0009-8291-1
10 ml

Heparin Sodium
Injection, USP

Sterile Solution from beef lung

5,000 Units per ml

For subcutaneous or intravenous use

NDC 0009-8291-1
4 ml

Heparin Sodium
Injection, USP

Sterile Solution

10,000 Units per ml

from beef lung

For subcutaneous or intravenous use

---

a. A patient is to receive 4,000 units of heparin by SC injection. How much
of the 5,000 units per ml solution should the patient receive?   _____

b. A patient is to receive 3,000 units of heparin by SC injection. How much
of the 10,000 units per ml solution should the patient receive?   _____

c. A patient is to receive 600 units of heparin by SC injection. How much of
the 1,000 units per ml solution should the patient receive?   _____

d. A patient is to receive 7,500 units of heparin by SC injection. How much
of the 10,000 units per ml solution should the patient receive?   _____

e. A patient is to receive 950 units of heparin by SC injection. Which of the 3 strengths shown would allow the person injecting the drug to measure it most accurately in a tuberculin syringe?

_____

f. A patient is to receive 1,250 units of heparin by SC injection. Which of the 3 strengths shown could be used to administer the ordered dose with the smallest amount of solution used?

_____

Unit 46 CALCULATING DOSAGE BY WEIGHT

BASIC PRINCIPLES OF CALCULATING DOSAGE BY WEIGHT

Many medications are calculated by body weight to obtain an accurate dosage based on the size of the individual taking the medication. Since average medication dosages are based on the body size of an average adult, this could mean an excess amount for a child or small adult or an insufficient amount for a very large adult. Package inserts provided with medications or the *Physician's Desk Reference* provide information based on body weight. For example, the recommended dose of Tetracycline, an antibiotic, is 25 mg/kg/day. This can be interpreted to read that for every kilogram of body weight the person should receive 25 milligrams of the medication per day. To calculate the correct dosage, weight must first be converted to kilograms. The weight in kilograms is then multiplied by the unit of measurement recommended per kilogram. The product is then divided by the number of doses per day to obtain the correct dosage of medication to give at one time.

Example: A 66-pound (lb) child is to receive 25 mg/kg/day of tetracycline tid (three times a day). Tetracycline is available in 100-mg and 250-mg capsules.

First convert the weight in pounds to kilograms:

1 kilogram (kg) = 2.2 pounds (lb)   This is the correct metric conversion factor.

$$\frac{2.2\ lb}{1\ kg} = \frac{66\ lb}{X\ kg}$$ Set up a proportion with the known fact.

$2.2 \times X = 2.2X$ Multiply the extremes.

$1 \times 66 = 66$ Multiply the means.

$2.2X = 66$ Write as means equals extremes.

$$\frac{2.2X}{2.2} = \frac{66}{2.2}$$ Divide both sides by 2.2 to find X

$X = 30\ kg$ The child weighs 30 kg.

Then set up a proportion to determine the recommended daily dosage: (Remember that the recommended dosage is 25 mg per kg per day.)

$$\frac{25\ mg}{1\ kg} = \frac{X\ mg}{30\ kg}$$ Set up a proportion with the known fact.

$25 \times 30 = 750$ Multiply the extremes.

$1 \times X = 1X$ Multiply the means.

$1X = 750$ Write as means equals extremes.

$$\frac{1X}{1} = \frac{750}{1}$$ Divide both sides by 1 to find X

$X = 750\ mg$ The recommended daily dosage is 750 mg.

Next, divide the total daily dosage by the number of doses to be given in a one-day period:

The order is for tid or three doses per day.

750 mg/3 = 250 mg per dose

Finally, use the proportion method or formula method to calculate the correct dose: Since 250 mg capsules are available, use them.

$$\frac{Known\ dosage\ available}{Known\ dosage\ form} = \frac{Dosage\ ordered}{Amount\ to\ be\ given}$$

$$\frac{250\ mg}{1\ cap} = \frac{250\ mg}{X\ cap}$$ (X is unknown.)

250 mg $\times$ X capsules = 1 capsule $\times$ 250 mg

$250X = 250$ (Divide both sides by 250.)

$250X/250 = 250/250$

$X = 1$ The correct dosage is 1 capsule.

At times, numbers must be rounded off to get the basic dosage. For example, if the child in the example weighed 50 pounds, this would equal 22.73 kg. Multiplying the 22.73 by the 25 mg/kg would equal 568.25 mg per day. Dividing by 3 to get the individual dose would result in a dose of 189.42. Since capsules cannot be cut or divided, it would be best to round the dose off to 200 mg per dose and give two 100-mg capsules for each dose.

PRACTICAL PROBLEMS

1. The recommended dose for meperidine is 6 mg/kg/day for pain. A child weighing 88 pounds can receive the medication q4h (every four hours).

   a. How many mg can the child receive per day?   _____

   b. How many mg can the child receive per dose? (*Hint:* Divide 24 hours by 4 hours to find the total number of doses per day.)   _____

2. The recommended dose for sulfasalazine, an antibiotic, is 30 mg/kg/day. An individual weighing 110 pounds is to take the medication tid (3 times a day).

   a. How many mg can the individual receive per day? _____

   b. How many mg can the individual receive per dose? (*Hint:* Remember the medication is tid.) _____

3. A child weighing 44 pounds is to receive cefadroxil for a urinary tract infection q12h (every 12 hours). The recommended dose is 30 mg/kg/day.

   a. How many mg can the child receive per day? _____

   b. How many mg can the child receive per dose? _____

4. A physician orders the diuretic Lasix® 20 mg IV stat (immediately) for a patient who weighs 72 pounds. The vial of Lasix® available is labeled:

65004285	Sterile: For intramuscular or intravenous drip use
4 ml vial	Store at controlled room temperature prior to constitution. Do not use if solution is discolored.
LASIX® (furosemide) INJECTION IM/IV	
For Single Use Only 4 ml – 40 mg (10 mg/ml)	**Recommended Dosage:** 1 to 2 mg per kg q 6 to 8 hours until desired diuretic response is attained. Maximum dose should not exceed 6 mg/kg per day.
Federal Law prohibits dispensing without a prescription.	

   a. What is the recommended dosage range in mg for this patient? _____

   b. Is the dosage ordered within this recommended range? _____

   c. How many ml of Lasix® should be injected? _____

5. The recommended dose of Ancef® for severe infections is 100 mg/kg/day. An individual weighs 124 pounds and is to receive the medication IM qid (four times a day).

   a. How many mg can the individual receive per day? _____

   b. How many mg can the individual receive per dose? _____

6. The recommended dose of Vancocin® for a severe staphylococcal infection is 40 mg/kg/day. The individual weighs 246 pounds and is to receive the medication IV q6h (every 6 hours).

   a. How many mg can the individual receive per day? _____

   b. How many mg can the individual receive per dose? _____

7. The recommended dose of Rondomycin®, an antibiotic, is 10 mg/kg/day. A person weighs 132 pounds and gets the medication qid (four times a day). Rondomycin® is available in 150-mg capsules.

    a. How many mg can the individual receive per dose?   _____

    b. How many capsules should the person receive per dose?   _____

8. A physician orders 10 ml of the antibiotic Tegopen® for a child weighing 48 pounds. Read the label carefully.

NDC 0015-7941-40 100 ml bottle **TEGOPEN®** CLOXACILLIN SODIUM FOR ORAL SOLUTION Equivalent to **125** mg per 5 ml when reconstituted according to directions. **Caution:** Federal Law prohibits dispensing without a prescription.	**Reconstitution:** Add a total of 63 ml of water to the bottle. Shake well. Bottle then contains 100 ml of solution. Each 5 ml contains cloxacillin sodium equivalent to 125 mg cloxacillin. **Usual Dosage:** Adults: 250 mg q6h Children: 50 mg/kg/day divided into even doses at 6-hour intervals. **Read accompanying circular**

    a. What is the maximum dose in mg the child can receive every day?   _____

    b. How many mg will the child receive if she gets 10 ml of solution?   _____

    c. What is the total dosage in mg if she gets the medication q6h?   _____

9. The recommended dose of the antibiotic ampicillin® is 50 mg/kg/day. A child weighs 66 pounds and receives the medication q8h. Ampicillin suspension is available as 250 mg per 5 ml.

    a. How many mg should the child receive per dose?   _____

    b. How many ml should the child receive per dose?   _____

10. The recommended dose of kanamycin to treat tuberculosis is 15 mg/kg/day for an IM injection. A patient weighs 220 pounds and is to receive an IM injection q12h (every 12 hours). Kanamycin for injection contains 500 mg per 2 ml.

    a. How many mg should the patient receive per injection?   _____

    b. How many ml should the patient receive per injection?   _____

11. The recommended dose for the antibacterial medication Gantrisin® is 150 mg/kg/day. An infant weighs 22 pounds and gets the medication q4h.

> **Pediatric Suspension & Syrup**
>
> ## *GANTRISIN®*
> *Acetyl Sulfisoxazole/Roche*
>
> **0.5 Gram per 5 ml**

   a. How many mg of medication does the infant receive per dose?   _____

   b. How many ml of medication does the infant receive per dose? (*Hint:* All units of measurement must be the same. Convert 0.5 gm to mg.)   _____

12. The recommended dose for Chloromycetin®, an antibacterial medication for serious infections such as meningitis, is 50 mg/kg/day in 4 equally divided doses. A patient weighs 176 pounds and is to receive the medication q6h. Chloromycetin® is available as 0.25 gm capsules.

   a. How many mg should the patient receive per dose?   _____

   b. How many capsules should the patient receive per dose?   _____

13. The recommended dose for the antifungal agent Ancobon® is 50 to 150 mg/kg/day administered q6h. It is available in 250-mg capsules. A patient weighs 162 pounds.

   a. What is the range in mg the patient could take per dose?   _____

   b. What is the range in number of capsules the patient could take per dose?   _____

14. A physician orders a dose of 0.125 mg of Lanoxin® elixir q12h for a 3-year-old child with a heart condition. The child weighs 36 pounds. Read the label carefully.

NDC 0173-0264-27 60 ml **LANOXIN®** (DIGOXIN) Pediatric Elixir Each ml contains **0.05 mg** **Caution:** Federal Law prohibits dispensing without a prescription.	Alcohol 10%, Methylparabyn 0.1% (added as preservative) Store at 15° to 25°C (59° to 77°F) and protect from sunlight. **Recommended Digitalization Dosage:** Adults: 0.75–1.25 mg per day and given at 6–8 hour intervals 5–10 Years: 0.02–0.035 mg/kg/day 2–5 Years: 0.03–0.05 mg/kg/day 1 Month–2 Years: 0.035–0.06 mg/kg/day

a. What is the range for the recommended dose in mg? _____

b. Is the dosage ordered within the recommended range? _____

c. How many ml should the child receive per dose? _____

15. The recommended dose for aminophylline, a bronchodilator used to treat asthma, is 12 mg/kg/day divided into 4 equal doses. It is available as 100-mg tablets. A child weighs 41 pounds.

a. How many mg should the child receive per dose? _____

b. How many tablets should be given per dose? (*Hint:* Remember it is necessary to round off to a reasonable size tablet.) _____

16. A child has pinworms. The recommended dose for Mintezol® suspension is 0.01 gm/kg/day given bid (2 times per day) after meals (pc). It is available as 500 mg per 5 ml. A child weighs 39 pounds.

a. What is the maximum dose in mg that can be given per dose? (*Hint:* Remember all units of measurement must be the same.) _____

b. If the maximum dose is given to the child, how many ml should be given per dose? _____

17. The recommended adult dose for streptomycin, an antibiotic, is 15 to 25 mg/kg/qd. A person weighing 94 pounds is to receive 2 ml injected every 8 hours.

> **5 ml Multiple Dose Vial**
>
> ## *STREPTOMYCIN SULFATE*
> *For IM Use*
>
> **1 Gram per 5 ml**

   a. Is the injection ordered within the recommended dosage?   _____

   b. How many mg will the patient receive per day?   _____

18. The recommended dose for theophylline, used to treat asthma by dilating the bronchi, is 5–6 mg/pound/day given twice a day. It is available as 200-mg tablets. How many tablets should a 156 pound person take per day?   _____

19. The recommended adult dose for midazolam is 0.07 to 0.08 mg/kg IM one hour before surgery to relax the patient. It is available as 5 mg per ml and must be given in exact dosage. How many ml should be injected into a 182-pound patient? Round off to nearest one-tenth of a ml.   _____

20. A patient has a severe fungal infection. She has good heart and kidney function and weighs 141 pounds. The physician orders 2 ml of Fungizone® to be infused over 4 hours IV bid (twice a day) on the first day. On day two, the dose is increased to 3 ml IV bid. On day three, the dose is increased to 4 ml bid.

NDC 0449-8668-522

10 ml

FUNGIZONE®
Amphotericin B for Injection USP

5 mg per ml

Dosage and Administration

Caution: Under no circumstances should a total daily dose of 1.5 mg/kg be exceeded. Amphotericin B overdoses can result in cardio-respiratory arrest.
In patients with good cardi-renal function and a well tolerated test dose, therapy is usually initiated with a daily dose of 0.25 mg/kg of body weight. Depending on the patient's status, doses may gradually be increased by 5 to 10 mg per day to a final daily dosage of 0.5 to 0.7 mg/kg.

a. How many mg of medication will the patient receive on day 1?   _____

b. Is this dosage within the recommended initial therapy dose? Why or why not?   _____

c. How many mg can the patient receive on day 2?   _____

d. Is the dose ordered for day 2 within the recommended amount? Why or why not?   _____

e. How many ml can the patient receive on day 3?   _____

f. Is the dose ordered for day 3 within the recommended amount? Why or why not?   _____

g. If you were the person who was to administer this medication, would you give it to the patient? Why or why not?   _____

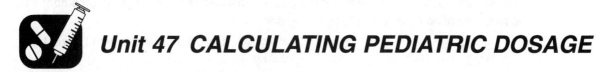

Unit 47 CALCULATING PEDIATRIC DOSAGE

BASIC PRINCIPLES OF CALCULATING PEDIATRIC DOSAGE

Correct medication dosages for infants and children are based on weight, height, body surface area, and age. An accurate dose is usually a fraction of the amount of medication given to an adult. It is extremely important to calculate the dosage accurately. A minor error in calculating dosage for an infant or child can be extremely serious, causing an overdose and even death. The person administering a medication to an infant or child must always make sure that the dose is safe according to the manufacturer's instructions. Thre are only two acceptable ways to determine pediatric dosage: calculating dosage based on kilograms or pounds of body weight and calculating dosage based on body surface area (BSA).

Calculation of Dosage Based on Body Weight:

Most drug manufacturers and medication reference books such as the *Physician's Desk Reference* (PDR) provide a recommended pediatric dosage based on kilograms of body weight. The infant or child must be weighed. Usually weight is recorded in pounds and ounces or pounds and fractions of pounds. The pounds must first be converted to kilograms. Then dosage can be calculated based on the number of kilograms the infant or child weighs.

Example: A physician orders acetaminophen 125 q4h (every four hours) for an infant with a high fever. The safe dosage range for acetaminophen is 10–15 mg/kg q4h. The infant weighs $22\frac{1}{2}$ pounds (lb). Is this a safe dose for the infant?

First convert the infant's weight in pounds to kilograms.

A known fact is that 1 kg = 2.2 lb.

$\dfrac{2.2 \text{ lb}}{1 \text{ kg}} = \dfrac{22.5 \text{ lb}}{X \text{ kg}}$	Set up a proportion with the known fact.
$2.2 \times X = 2.2X$	Multiply the extremes.
$1 \times 22.5 = 22.5$	Multiply the means.
$2.2X = 22.5$	Write as means equals extremes.
$\dfrac{2.2\ X}{2.2} = \dfrac{22.5}{2.2}$	Divide both sides by 2.2 to find X.
$X = 10.2272 \text{ kg}$	The infant weighs 10.2 kg.

Then set up a proportion to determine the recommended dosage range. (Remember that the recommended dosage is 10–15 mg/kg q4h.)

$$\frac{10 \text{ mg}}{1 \text{ kg}} = \frac{X \text{ mg}}{10.2 \text{ kg}} \qquad \frac{15 \text{ mg}}{1 \text{ kg}} = \frac{X \text{ mg}}{10.2 \text{ kg}} \qquad \text{Set up proportions with known facts.}$$

$10 \times 10.2 = 102$	$15 \times 10.2 = 153$	Multiply the extremes.
$1 \times X = 1X$	$1 \times X = 1X$	Multiply the means.
$1X = 102$	$1X = 153$	Write as means equals extremes.
$\dfrac{1X}{1} = \dfrac{102}{1}$	$\dfrac{1X}{1} = \dfrac{153}{1}$	Divide both sides by 1 to find X
$X = 102 \text{ mg}$	$X = 153 \text{ mg}$	Dosage range is 102–153 mg q4h.

The ordered dosage of 125 mg q4h would be a safe dosage for this infant.

Calculation of Dosage Based on Body Surface Area (BSA):

Pediatric dosage can also be calculated by using body surface area or BSA. The BSA method is considered to be one of the most accurate methods of calculating dosages since it relies on both the height and weight of the child. A nomogram is used to determine the BSA.

To determine BSA, the height of the child in inches (in) or centimeters (cm) is located on the left column of the nomogram. The weight of the child in kilograms (kg) or pounds (lb) is located on the right column. A straight edge, such as a ruler, is used to connect the two points. The point of intersection on the middle column provides the BSA in m² (meters squared). The example drawn on the nomogram shows a height of 35 inches and a weight of 30 pounds resulting in a BSA of 0.6 m². This BSA can then be inserted into a formula that uses a BSA of 1.7 m² for the average adult dosage.

Example: The usual adult dose for Demerol® is 50 mg per ml IM. A child is 35 inches (in) tall and weighs 30 pounds (lb). What is the correct dosage of Demerol® for this child? (*Note:* BSA on nomogram is 0.6 m² for this child.)

$$\text{Child's Dose} = \frac{\text{BSA of child in m}^2}{1.7 \text{ m}^2 \text{ (Adult average)}} \times \text{Adult dose}$$

$$\text{Child's Dose} = \frac{0.6 \text{ m}^2}{1.7 \text{ m}^2} \times 50 \text{ mg}$$

$$\text{Child's Dose} = 0.3529 \times 50 = 17.65 \text{ mg}$$

The correct dose of Demerol® for this child is 17.65 mg, usually rounded off to 18 mg.

Since Demerol® is provided as 50 mg per ml, the dosage must be calculated in ml.

$$\frac{50 \text{ mg}}{1 \text{ ml}} \diagdown\kern-1em=\kern-1em\diagup \frac{18 \text{ mg}}{X \text{ ml}}$$ Set up a proportion to calculate dosage.

$50 \times X = 50X \qquad 1 \times 18 = 18$ Multiply the means and extremes.

$50X = 18$ Write as means equals extremes.

$$\frac{50}{50} = \frac{18}{50}$$ Divide both sides by 50 to find X.

$X = 0.36 \text{ ml}$ Dosage would be 0.36 ml IM.

The formula above is based on an average adult with a mean body surface of 1.7. Some drugs, such as the medications used to treat cancer, must be calculated even more accurately. For this reason, many drug manufacturers now provide a recommended dose per m^2. This information is usually found in the page of instructions provided with every drug. The formula used to calculate dosage when this information is available is:

$$\frac{\text{Recommended average dose}}{1 m^2} = \frac{\text{Child's dose (unknown)}}{\text{Child's BSA } m^2}$$

Example: A physician orders methotrexate 25 mg IM for an 8-year-old girl with cancer. The manufacturer's recommended dose is 30 mg/m^2. The girl is 44 inches tall and weighs 55 pounds. Is 30 mg IM a safe dose for this girl?

Use a straight edge to connect the height of 44 inches and the weight of 55 pounds on the nomogram. It shows this child has a BSA of 0.9 m^2.

$$\frac{30 \text{ mg (recommended dose)}}{1 m^2} \diagdown\kern-1em=\kern-1em\diagup \frac{X \text{ (Child's dose)}}{0.9 m^2 \text{ (Child's BSA)}}$$

$1X = 30 \times 0.9$

$X = 27 \text{ mg}$ The child's dose is 27 mg.

The ordered dosage of 25 mg is safe for this child.

Methotrexate is available as 25 mg per ml, so the child would receive 1 ml.

WEST'S NOMOGRAM FOR ESTIMATION OF BODY SURFACE AREA (BSA)

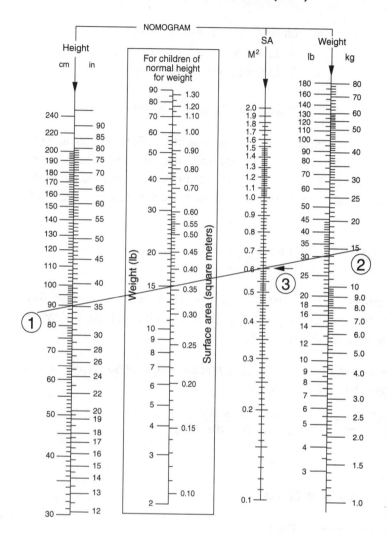

Body surface area (BSA) is determined by drawing a straight line from the patient's height ① in the far left column to his or her weight ② in the far right column. Intersection of the line with the body surface area (BSA) column ③ is the estimated BSA (m²). For infants and children of normal height for weight, BSA may be estimated from weight alone by referring to the enclosed area.

PRACTICAL PROBLEMS

1. A physician orders Vantin® 50 mg po (by mouth) q12h (every 12 hours) for an infant with a respiratory infection who weighs 22 pounds. The manufacturer recommends a dose of 5 mg/kg q12h.

    a. Is 50 mg a safe dose for the infant? _____

    b. If Vantin® is available in an oral suspension containing 50 mg/5 ml, how many ml would the infant receive per dose? _____

2. A physician orders aztreonam 500 mg IM tid (three times a day) for a child with a urinary tract infection. The child weighs 44 pounds. The manufacturer recommends a dose of 30 mg/kg q8h, not to exceed 120 mg/kg per day.

    a. Is 500 mg IM tid a safe dose for the child? _____

    b. What is the total dose in mg per day the child would receive? _____

    c. If aztreonam is available for injection as 1 gram per 2 ml, how many ml would be injected per dose? _____

3. Acetaminophen has a safe dosage range of 10 to 15 mg/kg q4h (every four hours). It is used as an antipyretic, or medication to reduce a fever. A 1-year-old child weighs 26 pounds.

    a. What is the safe dosage range in mg per dose of acetaminophen for this child? _____

    b. What is the maximum dose in mg per dose the child could receive in a 24-hour period? _____

4. A 15-month-old infant is scheduled for surgery. The infant weighs 18 pounds. The anesthesiologist orders Thorazine® 4 mg po (by mouth) 2 hours preop (before surgery) as a sedative. The literature states the dose should be 0.55 mg/kg q 4 to 6 hours.

> **120 Milliliters**
>
> ### *THORAZINE® SYRUP*
> *Chlorpromazine, U.S.P*
>
> **10 milligrams in 5 milliliters**

a. Is the ordered dosage safe for this infant?   _____

b. How many ml of syrup should be given to the infant if the ordered dosage is safe?   _____

5. A physician orders Prednisone Intensol Concentrate® Syrup 9 mg qid (four times a day) for a child with muscular dystrophy. The manufacturer recommends a dose of 0.75 to 1.5 mg/kg/day to improve muscle strength. The child weighs 56 pounds.

a. What is the safe range of dosage for this child?   _____

b. The prednisone syrup is available as 15 mg/5 ml solution. How many ml should the child receive per dose?   _____

c. How many mg will the child receive in a 24-hour period?   _____

6. A physician orders minoxidil 5 mg po (by mouth) qd (every day) for a 9-year-old child with hypertension or high blood pressure. The child weighs 76 pounds. The manufacturer recommends an initial dose of 0.2 mg/kg/day.

a. Is the dosage ordered a safe dose for this child?   _____

b. Minoxidil is available as 2.5-mg tablets. How many tablets should the child receive for the ordered dosage?   _____

7. A physician orders amoxicillin 400 mg po tid for child with strep throat. The child weighs 68 pounds. Read the label carefully.

NDC 0029-6009-21 80 ml (when reconstituted) **AMOXIL®** AMOXICILLIN For Oral Suspension 250 mg/5 ml **Caution:** Federal Law prohibits dispensing without a prescription.	**Directions for mixing:** Tap bottle until all powder flows freely. Add approximately 1/3 of a total of 59 ml of water for reconstitution. Shake vigorously to wet powder. Add remaining water and shake vigorously. Each 5 ml (1 teaspoon) will contain an equivalent of 250 mg amoxicillin. **Usual Adult Dosage:** 250 to 500 mg every 8 hours. **Usual Child Dosage:** 20 to 40 mg/kg/day in divided doses every 8 hours. See accompanying prescribing information.

   a. What is the recommended dosage range of amoxicillin for this child?   _____

   b. Is the dosage ordered safe for this child?   _____

   c. How many ml of Amoxil® should be given per ordered dose?   _____

   d. How many mg of Amoxil® will the child receive in a 24-hour period?   _____

8. A physician orders Rocephin® 100 mg/kg IV in divided doses q12h for a child with meningitis. The child weighs 53 pounds. The recommended dose is 100 mg/kg per day not to exceed a total dose of 4 grams (gm).

   a. What dose in mg should this child receive every 12 hours?   _____

   b. Does this dose meet the restriction of no more than 4 gm per 24 hours?   _____

   c. If Rocephin® is available at 1 gm/50 ml for injection, how many ml should be given to this child every 12 hours?   _____

Use the nomogram at the start of this unit to determine the correct BSA for problems 9 to 15.

9. An infant is 26 inches tall and weighs 22 pounds. What dose of Wycillin® should the infant receive if the adult dose is 600,000 U (units) qd (every day) IM. It is available as 600,000 U per ml for injection.

   a. How many U of Wycillin® should the infant receive?   _____

   b. How many ml should the infant receive? Round off to the nearest hundredth of a ml.   _____

10. A physician orders Demoral® 15 mg IM preop for a child scheduled for a tonsillectomy. The child is 85 cm tall and weighs 14 kg.

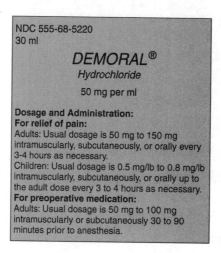

NDC 555-68-5220
30 ml

DEMORAL®
Hydrochloride
50 mg per ml

Dosage and Administration:
For relief of pain:
Adults: Usual dosage is 50 mg to 150 mg intramuscularly, subcutaneously, or orally every 3-4 hours as necessary.
Children: Usual dosage is 0.5 mg/lb to 0.8 mg/lb intramuscularly, subcutaneously, or orally up to the adult dose every 3 to 4 hours as necessary.
For preoperative medication:
Adults: Usual dosage is 50 mg to 100 mg intramuscularly or subcutaneously 30 to 90 minutes prior to anesthesia.

a. Is this a safe dose for the child?   _____

b. How many ml of Demerol® should the child receive?   _____

c. Shade the tuberculin syringe to indicate the dosage in ml that the child should receive. (*Hint:* Review Unit 32 on syringes.)

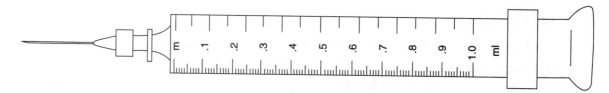

11. A child is 115 cm tall and weighs 30 kg. The normal adult dose for Diamox® tablets is 250 mg and it is available in 125-mg tablets.

a. How many mg should the child receive?   _____

b. How many tablets should the child receive? Round off to the nearest 1/4 tablet.

_____

12. An infant is 19 in tall and weighs 14 lb. The adult dose of Dilantin® is 100 mg. It is available in a pediatric form containing 30 mg per 5 ml.

a. How many mg should the infant receive?   _____

b. How many ml should the infant receive? Round off to the nearest tenth of a ml.

_____

13. A child is 105 cm tall and weighs 20 kg. The adult dose of Polymox® is 0.500 gm.

> **15 Milliliters**
>
> ### *POLYMOX® SUSPENSION*
> *Amoxicillin, U.S.P*
>
> **250 milligrams in 5 milliliters**

  a. How many gm should the child receive?   _____

  b. How many ml should the child receive rounded off to the nearest tenth of a ml? (*Hint:* All units of measurement must be the same.)   _____

14. A child is 35 in tall and weighs 42 lb. The maximum daily dose of Vistaril® is 400 mg for adults. It is available as a pediatric suspension containing 25 mg per 5 ml. If the child receives the medication qid (four times a day), how many ml should the child receive per dose? Round off to the nearest tenth of a ml.   _____

15. The recommended adult dose for lincomycin is 600 mg IM bid (twice a day). The injectable form contains 300 mg per 2 ml. An infant is 41 cm tall and weighs 4.5 kg.

  a. What is the total daily dose in mg that the infant can receive?   _____

  b. If the infant is injected q12h (every 12 hours), how many ml should be injected per dose? Round off to the nearest tenth of a ml.   _____

16. A physician prescribes Wellcovorin® 15 mg po q6h for a 15-year-old boy with colon cancer. The boy's BSA is 1.6 m^2. The manufacturer's recommended dose is 10 mg/m^2 po, IM, or IV q6h.

  a. Is the ordered dosage of Wellcovorin® safe for this boy?   _____

  b. What is the maximum dose this boy could receive per day?   _____

  c. If 5-mg tablets are available, how many tablets should he receive?   _____

17. An adolescent with Hodgkin's disease has a BSA of 1.4m². Her physician orders Blenoxane® IV. She has tolerated a test dose well with no reactions.

NSN 6505-01-060-4278
15 ml Vial

BLENOXANE®
(Sterile bleomycin sulfate, USP)

30 Units

Dosage and Administration:
Because of the possibility of an anaphylactoid reaction, lymphoma patients should be treated with two units or less for the first two doses. If no acute reaction occurs, then the regular dosage schedule may be followed.

Squamous cell carincoma, lymphosarcoma, testicular carcinoma: 0.25 to 0.50 units/kg (10 to 20 units/m²) given intravenously, intramuscularly, or subcutaneously weekly or twice weekly.

Hodgkin's Disease: 0.25 to 0.50 units/kg (10 to 20 units/m²) given intravenously, intramuscularly, or subcutaneously weekly or twice weekly.
After a 50% response, a maintenance dose of one unit daily or five units a week IV or IM should be given.

CAUTION: Pulmonary toxicity appears to be dose related with a striking increase when the total dose is over 400 units. Total doses over 400 units should be given with great caution.

   a. What is the dosage range for this patient?

   b. If Blenoxane® is available as 30 units per 15 ml of solution, how many ml of solution should the patient receive if the maximum dosage is administered intravenously?

18. A physician orders 1 teaspoon of Periactin® syrup tid (three times a day) for a child with allergies and rhinitis. The child's BSA is 0.76. The manufacturer recommends a dose of 8 mg/m² per day.

   a. What is the maximum dose in mg the child can receive per dose? (*Hint:* Remember the order states tid.)

   b. If Periactin® syrup is available as 2 mg per 5 ml, is the ordered dose safe for this child? Why or why not?

   c. How many mg will the child receive per day?

19. A 5-year-old boy has herpes simplex encephalitis. He has a BSA of 0.52m². The physician orders an intravenous infusion of Zovirax® 250 mg to be infused at a constant rate over 2 hours q8h (every 8 hours). The manufacturer recommends a dosage of 500 mg/m² infused at a rate over at least one hour q8h.

   a. What is the maximum dose in mg this boy can received per day?

   b. Is the ordered dosage safe? Why or why not?

20. An anesthesiologist orders Thorazine® 5 mg IM as a preop sedative for a child. The child has a BSA of 0.34 m². The manufacturer recommends a dose of 15 mg/m² 2 to 3 hours before surgery.

   a. What is the recommended dose of Thorazine® for this child?   _____

   b. Is the ordered dosage safe?   _____

   c. If Thorazine® for injection is available as 25 mg/ml, how many ml should be injected?   _____

   d. Shade the tuberculin syringe to show the correct dosage that must be administered to this child.

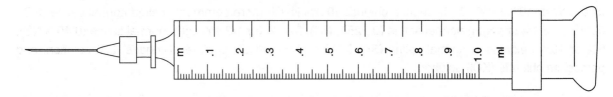

Unit 48 CALCULATING INTRAVENOUS FLOW RATES

BASIC PRINCIPLES OF CALCULATING INTRAVENOUS FLOW RATES

Intravenous (IV) fluids are fluids injected directly into a vein. They are used to replace body fluids or electrolytes, administer medications, or keep a vein open (KVO) for future use. There are many different types of IV fluids. Some of the most common ones include 5% or 10% dextrose (a form of sugar) in water (5% D/W or 10% D/W), 0.9% sodium chloride (0.9% NaCl) more commonly called normal saline (NS), 0.225% (or 1/4 strength) normal saline (0.225% NS), 0.45% (or 1/2 strength) normal saline (0.45% NS), 5% or 10% dextrose in normal saline (5% D/NS or 10% D/NS), Lactated Ringer's (LR) solution, and potassium chloride (KCl) solution.

A physician orders the type, amount, and flow rate for an IV solution or medication. The flow rate determines how much of the fluid enters the vein in a specific period of time. It is calculated as drops per minute (gtt/min).

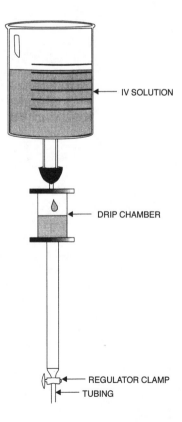

IV SOLUTION

DRIP CHAMBER

REGULATOR CLAMP

TUBING

IV infusion sets are used to regulate the flow rate. The sets contain intravenous tubing, a drip chamber, a regulator clamp to control the drip rate, and protective caps to maintain sterility. The label of every IV infusion set clearly states the drop factor or the number of drops per milliliter (gtt/ml) that the set is calibrated to deliver. There are two main types of drop factors in infusion sets: macrodrop and microdrop. A macrodrop infusion set may deliver 10 gtt/ml, 15 gtt/ml, or 20 gtt/ml depending on the manufacturer. A microdrop (or minidrip) infusion set delivers 60 gtt/ml no matter who the manufacturer is.

Calculating IV Flow Rates:

By knowing the drop factor, the amount or volume of IV solution, and the time period for infusion, the correct IV flow rate can be calculated. The flow rate is always calculated in drops per minute or gtt/min. The following formula can be used to calculate the flow rate.

$$\textbf{Flow Rate (gtt/min)} = \frac{\textbf{Volume (total amount to infuse)} \times \textbf{Calibration (drop factor in gtt/ml)}}{\textbf{Total Time in Minutes}}$$

The formula is usually abbreviated as:

$$F = \frac{V \times C}{T}$$

Example: The physician orders 1000 ml of 5% Dextrose in Water (D_5W) to be infused in 8 hours. The drop factor of the infusion set is calibrated at 20 gtt/ml. What is the flow rate in drops per minute?

$$\text{Flow Rate (gtt/min)} = \frac{\text{Volume} \times \text{Calibration (drop factor)}}{\text{Time in Minutes}}$$

The time factor of 8 hours must be changed to minutes for the formula:

1 hours : 60 minutes = 8 hours : X minutes

$1X = 8 \times 60$

$1X = 480$

$X = 480$ minutes

Substitute the correct information in the formula:

$$\text{Flow Rate} = \frac{1000 \text{ ml} \times 20 \text{ gtt}}{480}$$

$$\text{Flow Rate} = \frac{2000}{480} = 41.66$$

Flow Rate = 41.66 rounded off to 42 drops per minute

Calculating Infusion Time:

Another calculation that may have to be made regarding IVs is infusion time. Infusion time is the total time required for a specific volume of an IV solution to infuse at a given flow rate. By knowing the total amount or volume of IV to infuse, and the number of milliliters (ml) infusing per hour, it is easy to determine total infusion time.

Example: Calculate the infusion time for an IV of 1000 ml of D$_5$W infusing at 50 ml/hour.

$$\text{Infusion Time} = \frac{\text{Total volume to infuse}}{\text{ml/hour being infused}}$$

$$\text{Infusion Time} = \frac{1000 \text{ ml}}{50 \text{ ml}} = 20$$

Infusion Time = 20 hours

In some instances, only the volume to infuse, the drop factor, and the drops per minute are known. In these instances, additional steps must be followed to obtain infusion time.

Example: Calculate the infusion time for an IV of 1000 ml of D$_5$W infusing at 20 gtt/min. The drop factor is 10 gtt/ml.

First calculate the ml per minute by setting up a proportion with the known fact of the drop rate of 10 gtt/ml:

10 gtt: 1 ml $=$ 20 gtt : X ml

$10X = 20$

$X = 2$ ml

The IV is infusing at the rate of 2 ml per minute.

Next calculate the ml per hour (hr) by using 60 minutes for one hour to set up an equal proportion:

2 ml : 1 minute $=$ X ml : 60 minutes

$1X = 2 \times 60$

$1X = 120$

$X = 120$ ml

The IV in infusing at the rate of 120 ml per hour.

Now use the formula to determine infusion time:

$$\text{Infusion Time} = \frac{\text{Total volume to infuse}}{\text{ml/hour being infused}}$$

$$\text{Infusion Time} = \frac{1000 \text{ ml}}{120 \text{ ml}} = 8.3$$

Infusion Time = 8.3 hours or 8 hours and 18 minutes ($\frac{3}{10} \times 60$ min = 18 minutes)

Calculating IV Fluid Volume:

At times you will have to determine the volume of IV solution that will be absorbed in a specific period of time. By knowing the amount of time, the flow rate in gtt/min, and the calibration or drop factor in gtt/ml, you can determine how much IV solution will be absorbed in the specific period of time. The same formula used to calculate flow rate can be used to calculate IV fluid volume.

$$\text{Flow Rate (gtt/min)} = \frac{\text{Volume (total amount to infuse)} \times \text{Calibration (drop factor in gtt/ml)}}{\text{Total Time in Minutes}}$$

However, the formula must be reversed to read as follows:

$$\text{Volume (total amount infused)} = \frac{\text{Time (in minutes)} \times \text{Flow Rate (gtt/min)}}{\text{Calibration (drop factor in gtt/ml)}}$$

Example: A bag of 0.9% NS (normal saline) is infusing at the rate of 20 gtt/min. The infusion set is calibrated for a drop factor of 15 gtt/ml. How many ml of solution will infuse during an 8-hour shift?

First the time of 8 hours has to be calculated in minutes:

1 hour : 60 minutes = 8 hours : X minutes

$1X = 60 \times 8$

$X = 480$ minutes

Now insert the known information into the formula:

$$V = \frac{T \times F}{C}$$

$$V = \frac{480 \text{ minutes} \times 20 \text{ gtt/min}}{15 \text{ gtt/ml}}$$

$$V = \frac{9600}{15}$$

$V = 640$ ml   640 ml of the IV solution will infuse in the 8-hour period.

Automated Infusion Pumps:

In many health care agencies, IV solutions are regulated electronically by IV infusion pumps. The pumps are programmed for a specific flow rate. Alarms sound when this flow rate is interrupted. For example, a patient's change in position can sometimes interfere with the infusion of an IV solution. If the electronic pump cannot regulate the set flow rate, an alarm sounds. In this way, the infusion rate is controlled accurately at all times.

There are many different kinds of electronic infusion pumps. A common type is a *patient controlled analgesia (PCA)* pump. The device is used to administer pain medication to a patient, usually for postoperative (after surgery) or cancer pain. A prefilled syringe of pain medication is inserted into the PCA pump. When the patient experiences pain, he or she can press a control button so pain medication is infused in the IV. The PCAs have a "lock-out" time factor that limits the amount of pain medication a patient can received. This prevents an overdose of pain mediation. The pumps also keep a record of the number of times the patient has pushed the button and of the amount of pain medication the patient has received.

Most electronic infusion pumps require that the number of milliliters per hours be programmed into the keypad on the pump. For example, a physician orders 1000 ml 5% D/W (dextrose in water) to infuse in 8 hours. By dividing the 1000 ml by the number of hours or 8, the rate of 125 ml/hr can be calculated. This rate is then programmed into the keypad. The electronic pump then calculates the number of drops per minutes that will infuse 125 ml in one hour. The pump automatically adjusts the flow rate so the correct amount of IV solution is infused.

Before using any electronic infusion pump, a health care worker must have proper training in its use. In most states, only people authorized to administer medications are legally permitted to operate electronic infusion pumps. Every health care worker must always be aware of his or her legal responsibilities.

PRACTICAL PROBLEMS

Use the correct formulas to work the problems that follow.

1. A physician orders an IV of D_5W to run at 100 ml per hour. The drop factor of the infusion set is 10 gtt/ml. What is the flow rate? _____

2. An IV of Lactated Ringer's is to run at 50 ml per hour. The drop factor of the infusion set is 15 gtt/ml. What is the flow rate? _____

3. An antibiotic is mixed as 50 ml of IV solution. It is to infuse in 1 hour. The drop factor of the infusion set is 60 gtt/ml. What is the flow rate? _____

4. Calculate the flow rate for an IV of 500 ml of normal saline (NS) to be infused in 8 hours. The drop factor of the infusion set is 20 gtt/ml. _____

5. What is the flow rate for an IV of 1000 ml of 0.45% normal saline (NS) to infuse in 12 hours? The drop factor of the infusion set is 10 gtt/ml.   _____

6. A physician orders 2000 ml of Lactated Ringer's solution to infuse in a 24-hour period. The drop factor of the infusion set is 20 gtt/ml. What is the flow rate?   _____

7. An IV of 500 ml of dextrose in normal saline (D/NS) should be infused in 4 hours. The drop factor of the infusion set is 15 gtt/ml. What is the flow rate?   _____

8. A physician orders 2 pints of blood to be infused in 10 hours. The drop factor of the infusion set is 10 gtt/ml. What is the flow rate? (*Hint:* One pint is equal to 500 ml.)   _____

9. An antibiotic IV solution contains 20 ml of solution to be infused in 15 minutes. The drop factor of the infusion set is 60 gtt/ml. What is the flow rate?   _____

10. An IV containing heparin in 500 ml of NS is to infuse at 30 ml per hour. What is the infusion time?   _____

11. An IV containing Xylocaine® in 1000 ml of 5% dextrose in water is to infuse at 20 ml per hour. What is the infusion time?   _____

12. An IV containing heparin in 250 ml of NS is infusing at 40 drops per minute. The infusion set is a microdrop. What is the infusion time?   _____

13. Tetracycline is prepared in 50 ml of an IV solution. It is infusing at 30 drops per minute. The drop factor of the infusion set is 20 gtt/ml. What is the infusion time?   _____

14. A physician orders 1 pint of blood followed by 500 ml of NS. It is infusing at 60 drops per minute. The drop factor of the infusion set is 15 gtt/ml. What is the total infusion time for both solutions?   _____

15. The physician orders one pint of blood to infuse in 2 hours. This is to be followed by 1000 ml of NS to infuse at 30 drops per minute. The drop factor of the infusion set is 15 gtt/ml.

    a. What is the flow rate for the blood?   _____

    b. What is the total infusion time for the two IV solutions?   _____

16. A physician orders 40 ml of an IV solution containing ampicillin to run in 30 minutes with a microdrop infusion set. This is to be followed by 500 ml of NS to infuse at 50 drops per minute with an infusion set of 20 gtt/ml.

    a. What is the flow rate for the ampicillin solution?   _____

    b. What is the total infusion time for the two IV solutions?   _____

17. A 10% D/W solution is infusing at the rate of 30 gtt/min. The infusion set is calibrated for a drop factor of 20 gtt/ml. How many ml of the solution will infuse in 4 hours?   _____

18. The physician orders an IV solution of NS to infuse at the rate of 52 gtt/min. The infusion set is calibrated for a drop factor of 15 gtt/ml. How much of the solution will infuse during 2 1/2 hours?   _____

19. A solution of Lactated Ringer's is infusing at a rate of 28 gtt/min. The infusion set is calibrated for a drop factor of 10 gtt/ml. The physician has ordered that the Lactated Ringer's solution be replaced with 1000 ml of 0.45% NS at 12 noon. It is now 8:30 A.M. How many ml of Lactated Ringer's will infuse before the solution is discontinued.   _____

20. An IV of 5% dextrose in Lactated Ringer's is infusing at the rate of 12 gtt/min with an infusion set calibrated at 60 gtt/ml. The physician has ordered that the IV be discontinued at 10:30 P.M. It is now 5:45 P.M. How many ml of the solution will infuse before the IV is discontinued?   _____

21. A 1000 ml 10% D/NS IV was ordered to infuse over 8 hours at a rate of 22 gtt/min. The infusion set is calibrated at gtt/ml. After 4 hours, the nurse notices that 650 ml have infused instead of the 500 ml that should have infused. In order to regulate the IV, the nurse must recalibrate the gtt/min. What should the new flow rate be? (*Hint:* Calculate how much solution is left to infuse over the last 4 hours. Then calculate the new flow rate in gtt/min.)   _____

22. An IV containing 500 ml of KCl was to infuse over two hours. After 3/4 hour, only 200 ml of solution remains. The infusion set is calibrated at 15 gtt/ml. What should the new flow rate be?   _____

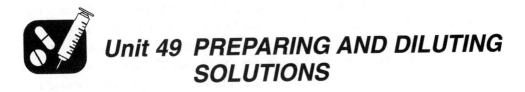

Unit 49 PREPARING AND DILUTING SOLUTIONS

BASIC PRINCIPLES OF PREPARING AND DILUTING SOLUTIONS

A solution is composed of two parts: a solvent and a solute. The solvent is the substance, usually a liquid, in which a substance is dissolved. The solute is the substance dissolved by the solvent.

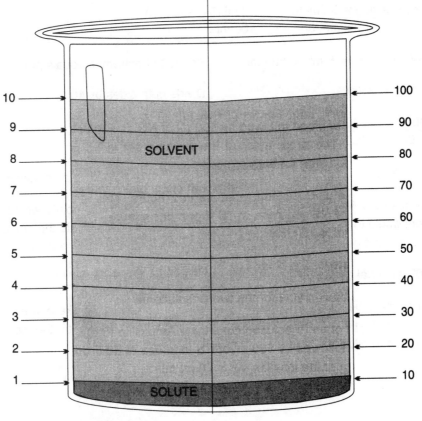

RATIO

1:10 SOLUTION

1 PART SOLUTE + 9 PARTS SOLVENT

TOTAL OF 10 PARTS

PERCENT

10% SOLUTION

10 PARTS SOLUTE + 90 PARTS SOLVENT

TOTAL OF 100 PARTS

The strength of solutions is stated as either a ratio or a percent. A solution with a ratio of 1:10 means that there is one part of solute in 10 parts of the solution. This means that one part of solute is mixed with 9 parts of solvent to equal a total of 10 parts. A 10% solution means that there are 10 parts of solute in 100 parts of the solution. This means that 10 parts of the solute are mixed with 90 parts of the solvent to equal a total of 100 parts. When both the solute and solvent are in liquid forms, both are expressed as milliliters (ml). A 1:10 boric acid solution is written as 1 ml/10 ml. A 10% boric acid solution is written as 10ml/100ml. When the solute is a solid and the solvent is a solution, the solute is expressed as grams (gm) and the solvent as milliliters (ml). A 1:20 dextrose solution is written as 1 gm/20 ml. A 5% dextrose solution is written as 5 gm/100 ml. These fractions are used to calculate the amount of solute that must be added to a solvent to prepare a solution.

Example: How many milliliters (ml) of boric acid solution are needed to prepare 500 (ml) of a 5% boric acid solution?

Calculate the boric acid in a 5% solution: 5 ml/100 ml

Set up a proportion: (Review Unit 22 if needed.)

$$\frac{X \text{ ml (Amount of solute)}}{500 \text{ ml (Total amount)}} = \frac{5 \text{ ml (5\% solution)}}{100 \text{ ml}}$$

$100 \text{ ml} \times X = 5 \text{ ml} \times 500 \text{ ml}$ Product of extremes equals product of means.

$100X = 2500$ Divide both sides by 100.

$$\frac{100X}{100} = \frac{500}{100}$$

$X = 25 \text{ ml}$ Use 25 ml of boric acid as a solute.

To prepare 500 ml of the 5% boric acid solution, 25 ml of the boric acid solute would be placed in a container. Solvent would then be added to total 500 ml of solution. To calculate the amount of solvent to add, subtract the amount of solute from the total quantity of solution desired:

500 ml (Total amount) − 25 ml (Solute) = 475 ml (Solvent)

At times, solutions must be diluted. A concentrated solution is used to make a weaker solution. The concentrated solution is used as the solute. A solvent is then added to the correct amount of concentrated solution to dilute the solution.

Example: How many milliliters (ml) of 5% boric acid solution are needed to prepare 100 ml of 5% boric acid solution?

Set up a proportion using the following formula:

$$\frac{\text{Desired strength}}{\text{Available strength}} = \frac{\text{Quantity of solute needed}}{\text{Total amount needed}}$$

Convert the strengths in percent to decimals:

5% = 0.05   25% = 0.25

Use the strengths expressed as decimals in the formula:

$$\frac{0.05}{0.25} = \frac{X \text{ ml (Unknown amount of solute)}}{100 \text{ ml (Amount of 5\% solution needed)}}$$

$0.05 \times 100 = 0.25 \times X$ Product of the extremes equals product of the means.

$5 = 0.25X$

$\dfrac{5}{0.25} = \dfrac{0.25X}{0.25}$ Divide both sides by 0.25 to final the value of *X*.

$20 = X$ Use 20 ml of the 25% boric acid solution.

To prepare 100 ml of a 5% boric acid solution, pour 20 ml of the 25% boric acid solution into a container. Subtract the amount of solute from the total amount desired to calculate the amount of solvent that must be added. In this case, subtract 20 ml from 100 ml to get 80 ml of solvent.

PRACTICAL PROBLEMS

1. How many milliliters (ml) of bleach are needed to prepare 100 ml of a 10% bleach solution? _____

2. How many ml of boric acid solution are needed to prepare 500 ml of a 1:5 boric acid solution? _____

3. How many grams (gm) of dextrose are needed to prepare 1000 ml of a 5% dextrose solution? _____

4. How many gm of sodium chloride (NaCl) are needed to prepare 600 ml of a 0.9% saline solution? _____

5. How many gm of sodium chloride (NaCl) are need to prepare 350 ml of a 0.225% saline solution? _____

6. A 750-ml bottle of solution is labeled 5% dextrose and 0.45% sodium chloride.

   a. How many gm of dextrose are in the bottle of solution?   _____

   b. How many gm of sodium chloride are in the bottle of solution?   _____

7. A 320-ml bottle of solution is labeled as a 7.5% bleach solution. How many ml of bleach are in the solution?   _____

8. How many ml of benzalkonium are needed to prepare one liter (l) of a 1:750 benzalkonium solution? (*Hint:* One liter is equal to 1000 milliliters.)   _____

9. How many ml of phenol are needed to prepare 250 ml of a 3% solution?   _____

10. Potassium permanganate tablets are available in one gram (gm) tablets. The tablets are used to prepare 400 ml of a 1:20 potassium permanganate solution.

    a. How many gm of potassium permanganate are needed?   _____

    b. How many tablets of potassium permanganate are needed?   _____

11. Sodium bicarbonate is available as 250-mg tablets. The tables are used to prepare 650 ml of a 1.5% sodium bicarbonate solution.

    a. How many gm of sodium bicarbonate are needed?   _____

    b. How many tablets of sodium bicarbonate are needed?   _____

12. Bichloride of mercury is available as 500 milligram (mg) tablets. The tablets are used to prepare 3½ liters (l) of a 1:1000 solution.

    a. How many gm of bichloride of mercury are needed?   _____

    b. How many tablets of bichloride of mercury are needed?   _____

13. How many ml of a 90% ethyl alcohol solution are needed to prepare 150 ml of a 70% ethyl alcohol solution?   _____

14. How many ml of a 1:750 benzalkonium solution are needed to prepare 500 ml of a 1:1000 benzalkonium solution?   _____

15. How many ml of a 6% acetic acid solution are needed to prepare 350 ml of a 2.5% acetic acid solution?   _____

16. How many ml of a 1:2 magnesium sulfate solution are needed to prepare 50 ml of a 15% magnesium sulfate solution?   _____

17. How many ml of a 23.5% sodium chloride (NaCl) solution are needed to prepare 750 ml of a 0.9% NaCl solution?   _____

18. How many ml of a 40% formaldehyde solution are needed to prepare 240 ml of a 1:25 formaldehyde solution?   _____

19. The label on a 500-ml bottle of Lactated Ringer's solution states that every 100 ml of solution contain the following solutes: 600 mg of sodium chloride, 30 mg of potassium chloride, 20 mg of calcium chloride, and 310 mg of sodium lactate.

    a. What is the percentage of sodium chloride in the solution? (*Hint:* Remember that percent is determined by the number of grams per 100 ml. Also remember that 1 gram is equal to 1000 milligrams.)   _____

    b. What is the percentage of potassium chloride in the solution?   _____

    c. What is the percentage of calcium chloride in the solution?   _____

    d. What is the percentage of sodium lactate in the solution?   _____

20. The label on a 50-ml bottle of 20 mEq (milliequivalents) potassium chloride solution states that each 100 ml contain 450 mg of sodium chloride, 5 gm of dextrose, and 149 mg of potassium chloride.

    a. What is the percentage of sodium chloride in the solution?   _____

    b. What is the percentage of dextrose in the solution?   _____

    c. What is the percentage of potassium chloride in the solution?   _____

21. Twenty ml of pure liquid cresol are added to 200 ml of solvent to form a solution. How many ml of the cresol solution would be needed to prepare 100 ml of a 2% cresol solution? (*Hint:* Calculate the percentage of the first cresol solution by creating a ratio or fraction.)   _____

22. Fifteen ml of pure bleach are added to 300 ml of solvent to form a solution. How many ml of the bleach solution would be needed to prepare 400 ml of a 1.5:500 solution?   _____

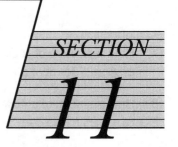

Introduction to Health Occupations

Unit 50 CAREERS IN HEALTH CARE

INTRODUCTION TO HEALTH CARE OCCUPATIONS

There are over 200 different occupations in health care. This section will provide a brief overview of some of these occupations, educational requirements, and average yearly salaries. Educational requirements use the following codes:

HOE: health occupations education program at the secondary (high school) or postsecondary (after high school) level

AD: Associate degree awarded by vocational-technical school or community college after completion of a prescribed course of study, usually two years in length

BD: Bachelor's degree awarded by a college or university after completion of a prescribed course of study, usually four years in length

MD: Master's degree awarded by a college or university after completion of one or more years of work beyond a bachelor's degree

DD: Doctorate or doctor's degree awarded by a college or university after completion of two to six years of study beyond a bachelor's or master's degree

Average yearly earnings are presented as a range of income, because earnings will vary according to geographical location, specialty area, level of education, and work experience.

Requirements for various health occupations can vary from state to state, so it is important for the student to obtain information pertinent to an individual state. Additional information about health occupations can be obtained from governmental publications such as the *Dictionary of Occupational Titles* and the *Occupational Outlook Handbook.* Both of these references also list other sources of information for each particular occupation. The internet is also an excellent source of information about the different health care occupations. Most of the occupations have professional organizations that provide detailed career information.

Dental Occupations:

Dentists are doctors who examine teeth and mouth tissues to diagnose and treat disease and abnormalities; perform surgery on the teeth, gums, and tissues; and work to prevent dental disease. Educational requirements are a DD, either DDS (doctor of dental surgery) or DMD (doctor of dental medicine). Average yearly salary is $84,000 to $200,000.

Dental hygienists work under the supervision of dentists. They perform preliminary examinations of the teeth and mouth, remove stains and deposits from the teeth, expose and develop X rays, and perform other preventive or therapeutic (treatment) services to help the patient maintain good dental health. Educational requirements are an AD or BD. Average yearly salary is $33,700 to $69,000.

Dental assistants work with the dentist or hygienist. They prepare patients for examinations, prepare dental materials, pass instruments and supplies, take and develop X rays, teach preventive care, sterilize instruments, and maintain the dental operatory. Educational requirements can be a HOE program or an AD. Average yearly salary is $15,600 to $31,200.

Dental laboratory technicians make and repair dentures, crowns, orthodontic appliances, and other dental prosthetics (artificial parts) according to the specifications of dentists. Educational requirements are a HOE program or AD. Average yearly salary is $19,400 to $52,600.

Diagnostic Services Occupations:

Cardiovascular technologists assist with cardiac catheterization procedures and angioplasty (a procedure to remove blockages in blood vessels), monitor patients during open-heart surgery and the implantation of pacemakers, perform tests to check circulation in blood vessels, and use ultrasound (high-frequency sound waves) to perform an echocardiograph. Educational requirements are an AD or BD. Average yearly salary is $27,500 to $53,200.

Electrocardiograph (ECG) technicians operate the electrocardiograph machine that records electrical impulses that originate in the heart, and perform stress tests (which record the action of the heart during physical activity), Holter monitorings (ECGs lasting 24 to 48 hours), thallium scans (a nuclear scan after thallium is injected), and other specialized cardiac tests that frequently involve the use of computers. Educational requirements are a HOE program or a special 6- to 12-month ECG program. Average yearly salary is $17,300 to $32,800.

Electroencephalographic (EEG) technologists perform diagnostic tests to record information on the electrical activity in the brain. Advanced training leads to a position as an *electroneurodiagnostic technologist.* These individuals perform nerve conduction tests, measure sensory and physical responses to specific stimuli, and operate other monitoring devices. Technologists who specialize in administering sleep disorder evaluations are called *polysomnographic technologists.* Educational requirements are a HOE program or an AD. Average yearly salary is $25,300 to $46,200.

Medical laboratory technologists (MTs), also called *clinical laboratory technologists,* examine tissues, fluids, and cells of the human body to help determine the presence and/or cause of disease. Specialty areas include biochemistry (chemical analysis of body fluids), cytotechnology (study of human body cells and cellular abnormalities), hematology (study of blood cells), histology (study of human cells and tissues), and microbiology (study of microorganisms causing disease). Educational requirements are a BD or MD. Average yearly salary is $33,500 to $55,200.

Medical laboratory technicians (MLTs) work with the medical technologist and perform many of basic medical laboratory tests. Educational requirements are a HOE program or AD. Average yearly salary is $25,700 to $33,500.

Phlebotomists or *venipuncture technicians* collect blood and prepare it for testing. Educational requirements are a HOE program or a 10- to 20-hour certification program. Average yearly salary is $12,800 to $26,300.

Radiologic technologists (RTs) work with X rays, radiation, nuclear medicine, ultrasound, magnetic resonance imaging (MRI), computerized tomography (CT), and positron emission scanners (PET) to diagnose and treat disease. Some specialty areas include *radiographers* who take X rays of the body for diagnostic purposes, *radiation therapists* who administer prescribed doses of radiation to treat diseases such as cancer, *nuclear medicine technologists* who prepare radioactive substances for administration to patients and then determine how the substances pass through the body, and *ultrasound technologists* or *sonographers* who use high-frequency sound waves to view different body organs. Educational requirements are an AD or BD. Average yearly salary is $28,900 to $51,400.

Biomedical equipment technicians (CBETs) work with the many different machines that are used to diagnose, treat, and monitor patients. Examples include patient monitors, kidney hemodialysis units, diagnostic imaging scanners, incubators for premature infants, electrocardiographs, X-ray units, pacemakers, artificial hearts, sterilizers, blood-gas analyzers, heart-lung machines, and respirators. They install, test, service, and repair the equipment, in addition to providing instruction on the correct use of the equipment. Educational requirements are an AD or BD. Average yearly salary is $22,500 to $52,400.

Emergency Medical Occupations:

Emergency medical technicians (EMTs) provide emergency, prehospital care to victims of accidents, injuries, or sudden illness. Levels of EMTs include the EMT ambulance/basic (EMT-B or EMT-1), the EMT intermediate (EMT-I, EMT-2, or EMT-3), and the EMT paramedic (EMT-P or EMT-4) and are achieved by the level of education completed. Educational requirements are approved EMT programs which begin with a minimum of 110 hours for EMT-B and expand to 2 years (over 1,000 hours) or an AD for EMT-P. Average yearly salaries depend on the level and average from $19,200 to $48,500.

Health Information and Communication Services:

Medical records (health information) administrators plan the systems for storing and obtaining information from records, prepare information for legal actions and insurance claims, compile statistics, manage medical records departments, ensure the confidentiality of patient information, and supervise and train other personnel. Educational requirements are a BD. Average yearly salary is $32,600 to $70,400.

Medical records (health information) technicians organize and code patient records, gather statistical or research information, and record patient information. Educational requirements are 30 semester hours of academic credit in medical records or an AD. Average yearly salary is $19,500 to $40,500.

Medical transcriptionists use a word processor to enter data that has been dictated on an audiotape recorder by physicians or other health care professionals. Examples include physical examination reports, surgical reports, consultation findings, progress notes, and radiology reports. Educational requirements are 1 or more years of a HOE program or correspondence courses. Average yearly salary is $14,500 to $29,900.

Unit secretaries, ward clerks, or *unit coordinators* are employed in hospitals, extended care facilities, clinics, and other health care agencies to record information on records, schedule procedures or tests, answer telephones, order supplies, and use computers to record or obtain information. Educational requirements are 1 or more years of technical education. Average yearly salaries are $14,200 to $34,300.

Medical illustrators use their artistic and creative talents to produce illustrations, charts, graphs, and diagrams for health textbooks, journals, magazines, and exhibits. Another related field is a *medical photographer* who takes photographs or records videotapes of surgical procedures, health education information, documentation of conditions before and after reconstructive surgery, and legal information such as injuries received in an accident. Educational requirements are a BD or MD. Average yearly salary is $35,000 to $65,200.

Medical librarians, also called *health science librarians,* organize books, journals, and other print materials to provide health information to other health care professionals. They use a computer to create information centers for large health care facilities. Some librarians specialize in researching information for large pharmaceutical companies, insurance agencies, lawyers, industry, and/or government agencies. Educational requirements are a MD. Average yearly salary is $35,000 to $136,300.

Hospital/Health Care Facilities Occupations:

Health care administrators manage the operation of health care facilities and are frequently called *chief executive officers (CEOs).* They hire and manage personnel, determine budget and finance, establish policies and procedures, perform public relations duties, and coordinate all activities in the facility.

Educational requirements are usually at least an AD or BD, and many positions require a MD or DD. Average yearly salaries depend on responsibilities and education but vary from $48,500 to $196,000.

Admitting officers/clerks work in the admissions department of a health care facility. They are responsible for obtaining all necessary information when a patient is admitted to the facility, assigning rooms, maintaining records, and processing information when the patient is discharged. Educational requirements are a HOE program or business/office technical education. Average yearly salary is $12,200 to $26,600.

Central/sterile supply technicians order, maintain, and supply all of the equipment and supplies utilized by other departments in a health care facility. They sterilize instruments and supplies, maintain all equipment, inventory materials, and fill requisitions from other departments. Educational requirements are a HOE program or on-the-job training. Average yearly salary is $12,200 to $23,500.

Medical Occupations:

Physicians or doctors examine patients, order tests, make diagnoses, perform surgery, treat diseases/disorders, and teach preventative health. Educational requirements are a DD such as a doctor of medicine (MD), doctor of osteopathy (DO), doctor of podiatric medicine (DPM), or doctor of chiropractic (DC). Many doctors specialize in specific fields of care. Average yearly salary is $120,000 to $305,000.

Physician's assistants (PAs) work under the supervision of the physician, take medical histories, perform routine physical examinations, do basic diagnostic tests, make preliminary diagnoses, and prescribe and administer appropriate treatments. Educational requirements are a minimum of a BD with an additional two or more years in a physician's assistant program. Average yearly salary is $38,600 to $83,200.

Medical assistants (MAs) prepare patients for examinations, assist with procedures and treatments, perform basic laboratory tests, prepare and maintain equipment and supplies, and assist the physician or physician's assistant. Educational requirements are a HOE program or AD. Average yearly salary is $15,200 to $33,400.

Mental and Social Services Occupations:

Psychiatrists are physicians who diagnose and treat mental illness. Educational requirements are a DD with additional years of study in psychiatry. Average yearly salary is $95,500 to $245,000.

Psychologists study human behavior and use this knowledge to help individuals deal with problems of everyday living. Some specialize in areas such as child psychology, adolescent psychology, geriatric psychology, behavior modification, drug/chemical abuse, and physical/sexual abuse. Educational requirements are a BD, MD, or even a DD for some positions. Average yearly salary is $24,900 to $71,800 or $38,900 to $92,500 with a doctorate.

Psychiatric/mental health technicians work with patients and their families to help them follow the treatment and rehabilitation plans established by the psychiatrist or psychologist. They provide understanding and encouragement, assist with physical care, observe and report behavior, and help teach patients constructive behavior. Educational requirements are an AD. Average yearly salary is $18,600 to $31,300.

Social workers or sociologists work with people who are unable to cope with various problems by helping them to make adjustments in their lives, and by referring patients to community sources for assistance. Educational requirements are a BD or MD. Average yearly salary is $28,600 to $56,800.

Mortuary Careers:

Funeral directors, also called *morticians* or *undertakers,* interview the family of the deceased to establish details of the funeral ceremonies or review arrangements the deceased person requested prior to death, prepare the body following legal requirements, secure information for legal documents, file death certificates, arrange and direct details of the wake and services, and direct all activities of the funeral home. Educational requirements are an AD or BD. Average yearly salary is $25,500 to $86,500.

Embalmers prepare the body for interment by washing the body with germicide soap, replacing the blood with embalming fluid to preserve the body, reshaping and restructuring disfigured bodies, applying cosmetics to create a natural appearance, dressing the body, placing the body in a casket, and maintaining embalming reports. Educational requirements are an AD or BD. Average yearly salary is $20,200 to $69,200.

Mortuary assistants work under the supervision of the funeral director and/or embalmer. They may assist with the preparation of the body, drive the hearse to pick up the body after death or take it to the burial site, arrange flowers for the viewing, assist with preparations for the funeral service, help with filing and maintenance of records, and clean the funeral home. Educational requirements are 1 to 2 years of on-the-job training or a HOE program. Average yearly salary is $12,200 to $25,800.

Nursing Occupations:

Registered nurses (RNs) provide total care to patients by observing patients, assessing patients' needs, reporting to other health care personnel, administering prescribed medications and treatments, teaching health care, and supervising other nursing personnel. Educational requirements are an AD, diploma, or BD from an accredited school of nursing. Specialties requiring additional education, such as a MD or DD, include nurse practitioners (CRNPs), nurse midwives (CNMs), nurse educators, and nurse anesthetists. Average yearly salary is $28,900 to $69,200 and may range from $60,300 to $108,900 with advanced specialties.

Licensed practical/vocational nurses (LPNs/LVNs) provide patient care that requires technical knowledge but not the depth of education of the registered nurse. Educational requirements are a 1- to 2-year state-approved practical/vocational nurse program. Average yearly salary is $23,200 to $43,100.

Nurse assistants, also called *nurse aides, nurse technicians, patient care technicians (PCTs),* and *orderlies,* work under the supervision of the RN or LPN/LVN and provide basic patient care. Specialties include geriatric assistants, who work with the elderly, and home health care assistants, who provide care in the home. Educational requirements are a state-approved HOE program. Average yearly salary is $14,000 to $27,200.

Surgical technicians/technologists (CSTs), also called *operating room technicians,* prepare patients for surgery; set up the operating room with instruments, equipment, and sterile supplies; assist during surgery by passing instruments and supplies to the surgeon; and provide postoperative care. Educational requirements may include a HOE program or an AD. Average yearly salary is $22,800 to $40,200.

Nutrition and Dietary Services:

Dietitians (RDs) manage food service systems, assess patient's nutritional needs, plan menus, teach others proper nutrition and special diets, purchase food and equipment, enforce sanitary and safety rules, and supervise other personnel. Educational requirements are a BD or MD. Average yearly salary is $28,000 to $59,600.

Dietetic technicians (DTs) work under the supervision of the dietitian and plan menus, order food, standardize and test recipes, assist with food preparation, and provide basic dietary instruction. Educational requirements are an AD. Average yearly salary is $20,200 to $46,200.

Dietetic assistants, also called *food service workers,* work under the supervision of dietitians and assist with food preparation and service, help patients select menus, clean work areas, and assist other dietary workers. Educational requirements are 6 to 12 months of on-the-job training or technical education. Average yearly salary is $12,200 to $21,000.

Therapeutic Services Occupations:

Occupational therapists (OTs) help people with physical, developmental, mental, or emotional disabilities to overcome, correct, or adjust to their particular problem by using various activities to assist a person in learning activities of daily living (ADL), adapting job skills, or preparing for return to work. Educational requirements are a BD or MD. Average yearly salary is $38,900 to $87,500.

Occupational therapy assistants/technicians (OTAs) help the patient carry out the program of treatment prescribed by the occupational therapist. They supervise arts and crafts projects, social events, recreational events, and therapeutic treatments. Educational requirements are a HOE program or an AD. Average yearly salary is $20,800 to $49,200.

Pharmacists dispense medications on written orders from physicians, dentists, and other health care professionals authorized to prescribe medications. They provide information on drugs, order and dispense other health care items, recommend nonprescription items to customers, ensure drug compatibility, maintain records, and supervise other pharmacy personnel. Educational requirements are a 5- to 6-year postsecondary degree in Pharmacy. Average yearly salary is $48,300 to $96,600.

Pharmacy technicians work under the supervision of a pharmacist and prepare medications for dispensing, label medications, perform inventories and order supplies, prepare intravenous solutions, and help maintain records. Educational requirements are a HOE program or an AD degree. Average yearly salary is $14,200 to $32,500.

Physical therapists (PTs) use exercise, massage, applications of heat/cold, water therapy, electricity, and/or ultrasound to provide treatment to improve mobility and prevent or limit permanent disability of patients with a disabling injury or disease. Educational requirements are a BD or MD. Average yearly salary is $42,500 to $89,600.

Physical therapy assistants/technicians (PTAs) work under the supervision of the physical therapist and carry out the prescribed plan of treatment. They perform exercises and massages; administer applications of heat, cold, and/or water; assist patients to ambulate with canes, crutches, or braces; provide ultrasound or electrical stimulation treatments; and inform therapists of the patients' responses and progress. Educational requirements are a 2-year accredited HOE program or an AD. Average yearly salary is $19,200 to $44,800.

Massage therapists use many variations of massage, bodywork (manipulation or application of pressure to the muscular or skeletal structure of the body), and therapeutic touch to muscles to provide pain relief for chronic conditions, improve lymphatic circulation to decrease edema (swelling), and release stress and tension. Educational requirements are a 3-month to 1-year accredited Massage Therapy program. Average yearly salary is $18,500 to $44,600.

Recreational therapists (TRs) use recreational and leisure activities as a form of treatment to improve the physical, emotional, and mental well-being of the patient. Activities might include organized athletic events, dances, arts and crafts, musical activities, field trips to shopping malls or other places of interest, movies, and poetry or book readings. Educational requirements are an AD or BD. Average yearly salary is $26,800 to $52,500.

Recreational therapy assistants, also called *activity directors,* work under the supervision of recreational therapists or other health care professionals. They assist in carrying out the activities planned by the therapists and, at times, arrange activities or events. Educational requirements are a HOE program or an AD. Average yearly salary is $13,500 to $32,800.

Respiratory therapists (RTs) treat patients with heart and lung diseases by administering oxygen, gases, or medications; using exercise to improve breathing; monitoring ventilators or respirators; and performing diagnostic respiratory function tests. Educational requirements are an AD or BD. Average yearly salary is $29,900 to $54,500.

Respiratory therapy technicians (RTTs) work under the supervision of respiratory therapists and administer respiratory treatments, perform basic diagnostic tests, clean and maintain equipment, and note and inform therapists of patients' responses and progress. Educational requirements are a 1- to 2-year HOE program or an AD. Average yearly salary is $19,800 to $34,500.

Speech-language therapists, also called *speech pathologists,* identify, evaluate, and treat patients with speech and language disorders to allow the patients to communicate as effectively as possible. Educational requirements are a MD. Average yearly salary is $33,200 to $80,500.

Audiologists provide care to individuals who have hearing impairments. They test hearing, diagnose problems, and prescribe treatment which may include hearing aids, auditory training, or instruction in speech or lip reading. They also test noise levels in workplaces and develop hearing protection programs. Educational requirements are a BD or MD. Average yearly salary is $33,200 to $80,500.

Art, music, and *dance therapists* use the arts to help patients deal with social, physical, or emotional problems. Educational requirements are a BD or MD. Average yearly salary is $21,200 to $56,800.

Athletic trainers (ATs) prevent and treat athletic injuries and provide rehabilitative services to athletes. They teach proper nutrition, assess the physical condition of athletes, give advice regarding a physical conditioning program to increase strength and flexibility or correct weaknesses, apply tape or padding on players to protect body parts, treat minor injuries, administer first aid for serious injuries, and help carry out any rehabilitation treatment prescribed by sports medicine physicians or other therapists. Educational requirements are a BD or MD. Average yearly salary is $22,400 to $58,600.

Dialysis technicians operate the kidney hemodialysis machine that is used to treat patients with limited or no kidney function. Educational requirements are a HOE program or an AD. Some states require RN or LPN licensure and state-approved dialysis training. Average yearly salary is $14,200 to $56,800.

Extracorporeal circulation technologists, also called *perfusionists,* operate the heart-lung machines used in coronary-bypass surgery. This field is expanding to include new advances such as artificial hearts. Educational requirements are a BD and specialized training that includes clinical experience. Average yearly salary is $36,200 to $64,500.

Veterinary Careers:

Veterinarians (DVMs or VMDs) are doctors who work with animals to prevent, diagnose, and treat diseases and injuries. Educational requirements are a DD in veterinary medicine. Average yearly salary is $39,500 to $92,800.

Veterinary technicians (VTs), also called *animal health technicians (ATRs),* assist with the handling and care of animals, collect specimens, assist with surgery, perform laboratory tests, take and develop X rays, administer prescribed treatments, and maintain records. Educational requirements are an AD or BD. Average yearly salary is $17,400 to $30,700.

Veterinary assistants, also called *animal caretakers,* feed, bathe, and groom animals; exercise animals; prepare animals for treatments; assist with examinations; clean and sanitize cages, examination tables, and surgical areas; and maintain records. Educational requirements are 1 to 2 years of on-the-job training or a HOE program. Average yearly salary is $13,200 to $21,300.

Vision Services:

Ophthalmologists are physicians who specialize in diseases and disorders of the eye. They diagnose and treat disease, perform surgery, and correct vision problems or defects, Educational requirements are a DD with a specialty in ophthalmology. Average yearly salary is $95,000 to $218,400.

Optometrists (ODs) examine eyes for vision problems and defects, prescribe corrective lenses or eye exercises, and in some states prescribe medications for diagnosis and/or treatment of eye disorders. Educational requirements are a DD from a college of optometry. Average yearly salary is $48,500 to $93,600.

Ophthalmic medical technologists (OMTs) obtain patient histories, perform routine eye tests and measurements, fit patients for contacts, administer prescribed treatments, assist with eye surgery, perform advanced diagnostic tests, administer prescribed medications, and perform advanced microbiological procedures. Educational requirements are an AD or BD. Average yearly salary is $23,000 to $38,600.

Ophthalmic technicians prepare patients for examinations, obtain medical histories, take ocular (eye) measurements, administer basic vision tests, maintain ophthalmic and surgical instruments, teach eye exercises, help patients with frame selection, order lenses, and teach proper care and use of contact lenses. Educational requirements are an AD. Average yearly salary is $20,100 to $27,600.

Ophthalmic assistants (OAs) prepare patients for examinations, measure visual acuity, perform receptionist duties, help patients with frame selections and fittings, order lenses, perform minor adjustments and repairs of glasses, and teach proper care and use of contact lenses. Educational requirements are a HOE program or specialized on-the-job training. Average yearly salary is $13,200 to $22,600.

Opticians make and fit the glasses or lenses prescribed by ophthalmologists and optometrists. Educational requirements are a HOE program or AD. Average yearly salary is $18,400 to $42,500.

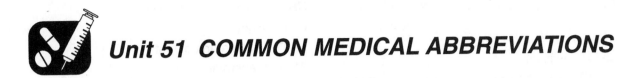

Unit 51 COMMON MEDICAL ABBREVIATIONS

Health care workers use a wide variety of medical abbreviations. Abbreviations are defined as shortened forms of words, usually just letters. Common examples include *AM,* which means morning, and *PM* which means afternoon or evening. Sometimes abbreviations are used by themselves. At other times, several abbreviations are combined to give orders or directions.

Example: 2 cap po qid q6h

This abbreviation gives a specific order for administering a medication.

It is interpreted as: 2 capsules by mouth four times a day every six hours.

As can be seen by the sample, it is much easier to write abbreviations than it is to write the corresponding detailed messages.

There is a growing trend toward eliminating periods from most abbreviations. Although the following list does not show periods, some health care agencies may use them. When in doubt, follow the policy of your agency.

The list that follows will provide a basic introduction to some of the most common abbreviations used in health care careers. It is essential that every health care worker be able to recognize and interpret these abbreviations.

@ — at

ac — before meals

AD — right ear

ADL — activities of daily living

ad lib — as desired

AIDS — acquired immune deficiency syndrome

AM, am — morning, before noon

amal — amalgam (dental restoration material)

AP — apical pulse

AS — left ear

ASA — aspirin

ASHD — arteriosclerotic heart disease

AU — both ears

Ax — axilla, axillary, armpit

bid — twice a day

Bl — blood

BM — bowel movement

BP — blood pressure

BR — bedrest

BRP — bathroom privileges

BS — blood sugar

BSA — body surface area

$\overline{c}$ — with

°C — degrees Celsius (Centigrade)

cal — calorie

Cap — capsule

CBC — complete blood count

cc — cubic centimeter

CDC — Centers for Disease Control and Prevention

CI — chloride or chlorine

cm — centimeter

COPD — chronic obstructive pulmonary disease

CPR — cardiopulmonary resuscitation

Cr — crown

C-section — Caesarean section, surgical removal of infant

CVA — cerebral vascular accident, stroke

dil — dilute

DNR — do not resuscitate

dr — dram, drainage

D/S — dextrose in saline

DW — distilled water

D/W — dextrose in water

ECG — electrocardiogram

EEG — electroencephalogram

EMS — emergency medical services

EMT — emergency medical technician

ESR — erythrocyte sedimentation rate

ext — extract, extraction, external

°F — degrees Fahrenheit

FBS — fasting blood sugar

FF or FFI — force fluids

ft — foot

gal — gallon

GB — gallbladder

GI — gastrointestinal

gm or g — gram

gr — grain

gtt or gtts — drops

GTT — glucose tolerance test

hct — hematocrit

Hg — mercury

hgb — hemoglobin

HIV — human immunodeficiency virus (AIDS virus)

Hr, hr, or h — hour, hours

HS — hour of sleep, bedtime

Ht — height

I & O — intake and output

ID — intradermal

IM — intramuscular

in — inch

inj — injection

IPPB — intermittent positive pressure breathing

IV — intravenous

K — potassium

KCI — potassium chloride

kg — kilogram

L or l — liter (1000 ml)

lb — pound

LPN — licensed practical nurse

m — minim

mcg — microgram

mcm — micrometer

MD — medical doctor

mEq — milliequivalent

mg — milligram

Mg — magnesium

min — minute

ml or mL — milliliter

mm — millimeter

MN — midnight

NaCl — sodium chloride

NG or ng — nasogastric (nose to stomach) tube

NPO — nothing by mouth

N/S or NS — normal saline

OD — right eye, occular dextro

OR — operating room

OS — left eye, occular sinistra

OT — occupational therapy

OU — each eye

oz — ounce

p̄ — after

P — pulse

pc — after meals

PCA —patient controlled analgesia

PDR — *Physician's Desk Reference*

pH — measure of acidity or alkalinity

PM, pm — after noon

po — by mouth, per orum

postop — after an operation

PP or pp — postpartum, after delivery

preop — before an operation

prn — whenever necessary, as needed

PT — physical therapy

pt — pint (500 ml or cc)

q — every

qd — every day

qh — every hour

q2h — every 2 hours

q3h — every 3 hours

q4h — every 4 hours

qhs — every night at bedtime or hour of sleep

qid — four times a day

qod — every other day

qoh — every other hour

qs — quantity sufficient

qt — quart (1000 ml or cc)

R — respiration or rectal

RBC — red blood cell or count

RDA — recommended daily allowance

RN — registered nurse

RT — respiratory therapist

Rx — prescription, take, treatment

s̄ or w/o — without

sc or SC — subcutaneous

Sig — give the following directions

Sol — solution

sos — if necesary

SpGr or sp gr — specific gravity

s̄s̄ — one half

SSE — soap solution enema

staph —staphylococcus infection

stat — immediately, at once

STD — sexually transmitted disease

strep —streptococcus infection

supp —suppository

Surg — surgery

T — temperature

tab — tablet

tbsp — tablespoon

tid — 3 times a day

TPR — temperature, pulse, and respiration

tsp — teaspoon

URI — upper respiratory infection

UTI — urinary tract infection

VS — vital signs (TPR and BP)

WBC — white blood cell or count

wt — weight

Symbols:

× — times (example: 2× means do two times)

> — greater than

< — less than

≠ — higher, elevate, up

ø — lower, down

— pound, number

℥ — dram

℥ — ounce

' — foot, minute

" — inch, second

° — degree

I or i — one

II or ii — two

V — five

X — ten

L — fifty

C — one hundred

D — five hundred

M — one thousand

Appendix

Section 1: METRIC AND ENGLISH LINEAR MEASUREMENTS

METRIC LINEAR (LENGTH/DISTANCE) MEASUREMENTS			
METRIC LINEAR UNIT	**SYMBOL**	**VALUE IN METERS**	**RELATION TO BASE UNIT**
kilometer	km	1,000.0 (10^3)	Multiply by 1,000
hectometer	hm	100.0 (10^2)	Multiply by 100
dekameter	dam	10.0 (10^1)	Multiply by 10
meter	m	1	Base Unit
decimeter	dm	0.1 (10^{-1})	Divide by 10
centimeter	cm	0.01 (10^{-2})	Divide by 100
millimeter	mm	0.001 (10^{-3})	Divide by 1,000

ENGLISH-METRIC LINEAR EQUIVALENTS				
		1 inch (in)	=	0.0254 meter (m)
12 inches	=	1 foot (ft)	=	0.3048 meter (m)
3 feet	=	1 yard (yd)	=	0.9144 meter (m)
5,280 feet	=	1 mile (mi)	=	1,609 meters (m)
39.372 inches	=	3.281 feet (ft)	=	1 meter (m)
		1.094 yards (yd)	=	1 meter (m)
		0.621 mile (mi)	=	1 kilometer (km)

Section 2: METRIC AND ENGLISH MASS OR WEIGHT MEASUREMENTS

METRIC MASS OR WEIGHT MEASUREMENTS			
METRIC MASS OR WEIGHT UNIT	SYMBOL	VALUE IN GRAMS	RELATION TO BASE UNIT
kilogram	kg	$1,000.0 \ (10^3)$	Multiply by 1,000
hectogram	hg	$100.0 \ (10^2)$	Multiply by 100
dekagram	dag	$10.0 \ (10^1)$	Multiply by 10
gram	gm or g	1	Base Unit
decigram	dg	$0.1 \ (10^{-1})$	Divide by 10
centigram	cg	$0.01 \ (10^{-2})$	Divide by 100
milligram	mg	$0.001 \ (10^{-3})$	Divide by 1,000

ENGLISH-METRIC MASS OR WEIGHT EQUIVALENTS
1 ounce (oz) = 0.028 kilogram (kg) or 28 grams (gm)
16 ounces (oz) = 1 pound (lb) = 0.454 kilogram (kg) or 454 grams (gm)
35.27 ounces (oz) = 1 kilogram (kg)
2.2 pounds (lb) = 1 kilogram (kg)

Section 3: METRIC AND ENGLISH VOLUME OR LIQUID MEASUREMENTS

METRIC VOLUME OR LIQUID MEASUREMENTS			
METRIC LIQUID OR VOLUME UNIT	**SYMBOL**	**VALUE IN LITERS**	**RELATION TO BASE UNIT**
kiloliter	kl	$1,000.0\ (10^3)$	Multiply by 1,000
hectoliter	hl	$100.0\ (10^2)$	Multiply by 100
dekaliter	dal	$10.0\ (10^1)$	Multiply by 10
liter	l	1	Base Unit
deciliter	dl	$0.1\ (10^{-1})$	Divide by 10
centiliter	cl	$0.01\ (10^{-2})$	Divide by 100
milliliter	ml	$0.001\ (10^{-3})$	Divide by 1,000

ENGLISH-METRIC VOLUME OR LIQUID EQUIVALENTS			
	1 drop (gtt)	=	0.0667 milliliter (ml)
	15 drops (gtt)	=	1.0 milliliter (ml)
	1 teaspoon (tsp)	=	5.0 milliliters (ml)
3 teaspoons =	1 tablespoon (tbsp)	=	15.0 milliliters (ml)
	1 ounce (oz)	=	30.0 milliliters (ml)
8 ounces (oz) =	1 cup (cp)	=	240.0 milliliters (ml)
2 cups (cp) =	1 pint (pt)	=	500.0 milliliters (ml)
2 pints (pt) =	1 quart (qt)	=	1000.0 milliliters (ml)

Section 4: METRIC, APOTHECARIES', AND ENGLISH EQUIVALENTS

METRIC-APOTHECARIES'-ENGLISH EQUIVALENTS		
APPROXIMATE METRIC	APOTHECARIES'	APPROXIMATE ENGLISH/HOUSEHOLD
Dry		
0.25 milligram (mg)	$\frac{1}{250}$ grain (gr)	
0.5 milligram (mg)	$\frac{1}{120}$ grain (gr)	
1 milligram (mg)	$\frac{1}{60}$ grain (gr)	
2 milligrams (mg)	$\frac{1}{30}$ grain (gr)	
4 milligrams (mg)	$\frac{1}{15}$ grain (gr)	
10 milligrams (mg)	$\frac{1}{6}$ grain (gr)	
15 milligrams (mg)	$\frac{1}{4}$ grain (gr)	
30 milligrams (mg)	$\frac{1}{2}$ grain (gr)	
45 milligrams (mg)	$\frac{3}{4}$ grain (gr)	
60 milligrams (mg)	1 grain (gr)	
100 milligrams (mg)	$1\frac{1}{2}$ grains (gr)	
500 milligrams (mg)	$7\frac{1}{2}$ grains (gr)	$\frac{1}{8}$ teaspoon (tsp)
1 gram (gm)	15 grains (gr)	$\frac{1}{4}$ teaspoon (tsp)
4 grams (gm)	1 dram (ʒ or dr) or 60 grains (gr)	1 teaspoon (tsp)
15 grams (gm)	4 drams (ʒ IV)	1 tablespoon (tbsp)
30 grams (gm)	8 drams (ʒ VIII) or 1 ounce (ʒ)	2 tablespoons (tbsp) or 1 ounce (ʒ)
360 grams (gm)	12 ounces (ʒ XII) or 1 pound (lb)	16 ounces (ʒ) or 1 pound (lb)
1 kilogram (kg)		2.2 pounds (lb)
Volume or Liquid		
0.06 milliliter (ml)	1 minim (m)	1 drop (gtt)
1 milliliter (ml)	15 minims (m)	15 drops (gtt)
4–5 milliliters (ml)	60 minims (m) or 1 dram (ʒ)	60–75 drops (gtt) or 1 teaspoon (tsp)
15 milliliters (ml)	4 drams (ʒ IV)	1 tablespoon (tbsp)
30 milliliters (ml)	8 drams (ʒ VIII) or 1 ounce (ʒ)	2 tablespoons (tbsp) or 1 ounce (oz)
500 milliliters (ml)	16 ounces (ʒ XVI) or 1 pint (pt)	16 ounces (oz) or 1 pint (pt)
1000 milliliters (ml)	2 pints (pt) or 1 quart (qt)	2 pints (pt) or 1 quart (qt)

Section 5: ROMAN NUMERAL EQUIVALENTS

ARABIC AND ROMAN NUMERAL EQUIVALENTS					
ARABIC	**ROMAN**	**ARABIC**	**ROMAN**	**ARABIC**	**ROMAN**
1	I	8	VIII	60	LX
2	II	9	IX	70	LXX
3	III	10	X	80	LXXX
4	IV	20	XX	90	XC
5	V	30	XXX	100	C
6	VI	40	XL	500	D
7	VII	50	L	1000	M

Section 6: FAHRENHEIT AND CELSIUS TEMPERATURE CONVERSIONS

To convert Fahrenheit (°F) to Celsius (°C):

$$C = (°F - 32) \times \tfrac{5}{9} \text{ or } C = (°F - 32) \times 0.5556$$

To convert Celsius (°C) to Fahrenheit (°F):

$$F = (°C \times \tfrac{9}{5}) + 32 \text{ or } F = (°C \times 1.8) + 32$$

COMMON CELSIUS/FAHRENHEIT CONVERSIONS					
°F	°C	°F	°C	°F	°C
32	0	101	38.3	114	45.6
70	21.1	102	38.9	115	46.1
75	23.9	103	39.4	116	46.7
80	26.7	104	40	117	47.2
85	29.4	105	40.6	118	47.8
90	32.2	106	41.1	119	48.3
95	35	107	41.7	120	48.9
96	35.6	108	42.2	125	51.7
97	36.1	109	42.8	130	54.4
98	36.7	110	43.3	135	57.2
98.6	37	111	43.9	140	60
99	37.2	112	44.4	150	65.6
100	37.8	113	45	212	100

Section 7: 24-HOUR CLOCK (MILITARY TIME) CONVERSION CHART

24-HOUR CLOCK (MILITARY TIME) CONVERSION CHART			
TIME	**24-HOUR TIME**	**TIME**	**24-HOUR TIME**
12:01 AM	0001	12:01 PM	1201
12:05 AM	0005	12:05 PM	1205
12:30 AM	0030	12:30 PM	1230
12:45 AM	0045	12:45 PM	1245
1:00 AM	0100	1:00 PM	1300
2:00 AM	0200	2:00 PM	1400
3:00 AM	0300	3:00 PM	1500
4:00 AM	0400	4:00 PM	1600
5:00 AM	0500	5:00 PM	1700
6:00 AM	0600	6:00 PM	1800
7:00 AM	0700	7:00 PM	1900
8:00 AM	0800	8:00 PM	2000
9:00 AM	0900	9:00 PM	2100
10:00 AM	1000	10:00 PM	2200
11:00 AM	1100	11:00 PM	2300
12:00 Noon	1200	12:00 Midnight	2400

Glossary

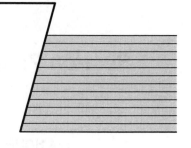

Acquired Immune Deficiency Syndrome (AIDS) — A disease caused by the HIV virus that attacks the body's immune system and causes the body to lose its ability to fight off infections and disease.

Agar — A gelatinous colloidal extract of red alga, used to provide nourishment for the growth of organisms.

Agglutination — The process of clumping together, as the clumping together of red blood cells.

Alginate — An irreversible hydrocolloid dental material used to take impressions of teeth or dental arches.

Amalgam — An alloy (mixture) of various metals with mercury; used as a restoration or filling material primarily on posterior (back) teeth.

Anatomy — The study of the structure of an organism.

Anticoagulant — A substance that prevents the clotting of blood.

Apical pulse — A pulse count taken with a stethoscope at the apex of the heart.

Appointment — A schedule to do something on a particular day and time.

Aquamatic pad — A temperature-controlled unit that circulates warm liquid through a pad to provide dry heat.

Axilla — The armpit; area of the body under the arms.

Bacteria — A group of one-celled micro-organisms; some are beneficial and some cause disease.

Bite-wing — A dental X ray that shows only the crowns of teeth; also called cavity-detecting X ray.

Blood pressure — A measurement of the force exerted by the heart against arterial walls when the heart contracts (beats) and relaxes.

Blood smear — A drop of blood spread thinly on a slide for microscopic examination.

Bowel movement (BM) — Elimination of indigestibles from the intestine through the rectum.

Caesarean section (C-Section) — A surgical operation done to deliver a baby by cutting through the mother's abdomen and uterus.

Cardiology — Study of the heart.

Cardiopulmonary resuscitation (CPR) — Procedure of providing oxygen and chest compressions to a victim whose heart has stopped beating.

Celsius (C) — A measurement scale for temperature on which 0° is the freezing point and 100° is the boiling point; also called centigrade.

Cement — A dental material used to seal inlays, crowns, bridges, and orthodontic appliances in place.

Centers for Disease Control and Prevention (CDC) — A division of the federal government that is concerned with causes, spread, and control of diseases in populations.

Check — A written order for payment of money through a bank.

Cholesterol — A fatty substance found in body cells and animal fat.

Composite — A dental restoration or filling material used most frequently on anterior (front) teeth.

Coronary — Pertaining to the heart or the arteries by the heart.

Culture specimen — A sample of micro-organisms or tissue cells taken from an area of the body for examination.

Deduction — Subtracted or taken out; amounts subtracted from a paycheck to pay for various things such as taxes.

Dental — Pertaining to the teeth.

Dental hygienist — A licensed individual who works with a dentist to provide care and treatment for the teeth and gums.

Dentist — A doctor who specializes in diagnosis, prevention, and treatment of diseases of the teeth and gums.

Deposit slip — A bank record listing all cash and checks that are to be placed in an account.

Dermatologist — A doctor specializing in diseases of the skin.

Diagnosis — Determining the nature of a person's disease.

Dialysis — Removal of urine substances from the blood by way of passing solutes through a membrane.

Dietitian — An individual who specializes in the science of diet and nutrition.

Differential count — A blood test that determines the percentage of each kind of leukocyte (white blood cell).

Electrocardiogram (ECG) — A graphic tracing of the electrical activity of the heart.

Electroencephalogram (EEG) — A graphic recording of the electrical activity in the brain.

Emesis — Vomiting; the expulsion of the contents of the stomach and/or intestine through the mouth and/or nose.

Endorsement — Writing a signature on the back of a check in order to receive payment.

Enema — An injection of fluid into the large intestine through the rectum.

Epidemiologist — An individual who researches and studies the cause of widespread outbreaks of a disease.

Erythrocyte — A red blood cell.

Erythrocyte sedimentation rate — A blood test that measures the rate at which red blood cells settle out of the blood.

Fahrenheit (F) — A measurement scale for temperature on which 32° is the freezing point and 212° is the boiling point.

Fasting blood sugar (FBS) — A blood test that measures the blood serum levels of glucose (sugar) after a person has had nothing by mouth for a period of time.

Feces — Waste material discharged from the bowels; also called stool.

Filing — To arrange in order.

Fungus — A group of simple plantlike animals that live on dead organic matter.

Geriatric — The study of the aged or old age and treatment of its diseases and conditions.

Glucose — The most common type of body sugar.

Gross pay — The amount of pay earned for hours worked before deductions are taken out.

Gynecology — The science of diseases of women, especially those affecting the reproductive organs.

Hemacytometer — A specially calibrated instrument with a measured and lined area for counting blood cells.

Hematocrit — A blood test that measures the percentage of red blood cells per given unit of blood.

Hematology — The study of the blood and blood diseases.

Hemoglobin — The iron-containing pigment of red blood cells that carries oxygen and gases from the lungs to the tissues.

Hemostat — An instrument used to compress (clamp) blood vessels to stop bleeding.

Hepatitis — An inflammation of the liver.

Histology — The study of the tissues and structure of tissues.

Hospice — Program designed to provide care for the terminally ill while allowing them to die with dignity.

Hypertension — High blood pressure.

Hypotension — Low blood pressure.

Impression — A negative reproduction of a tooth or dental arch; used as a mold to form a model of the tooth or dental arch.

Intake and Output — A record that notes all fluids taken in or eliminated by a person in a period of time.

Intradermal — Injected or put into the skin.

Intramuscular (IM) — To inject or put into a muscle.

Intravenous (IV) — To inject or put into a vein.

Ledger card — A card or record that shows a financial account of money charged, received, or paid out.

Legal —Authorized or based on law.

Leukocyte — A white blood cell.

Leukocyte count — A blood test that counts the total number of white blood cells per volume of blood.

Malignant — Harmful or dangerous; likely to spread and cause destruction and death.

Mandible — The horseshoe-shaped bone that forms the lower jaw.

Maxilla — The upper jaw bone.

Medication — A drug used to treat a disease.

Metabolism — The use of food nutrients by the body to produce energy.

Microbiology — The study of microscopic living organisms.

Microorganism — A small living plant or animal not visible to the naked eye.

Microscope — An instrument used to magnify or enlarge objects for viewing.

Miscarriage — The premature delivery of a fetus that results in the death of the fetus.

Model — A positive reproduction of the dental arches or teeth made out of plaster, stone, or another gypsum product.

Myocardial infarction — A heart attack; a reduction in the supply of blood to the heart with damage to the muscle of the heart.

Nasogastric tube — A tube inserted through the nose that goes down the esophagus to the stomach.

Neonatal — Pertaining to a newborn infant.

Net income — The amount of pay received for hours worked after all deductions have been taken out; take-home pay.

Neurology — The study of the nervous system.

Obstetrics — The branch of medicine dealing with pregnancy and childbirth.

Occupational therapy — Treatment directed at preparing a person requiring rehabilitation for a trade or for returning to the activities of daily living (ADL).

Oncology — The branch of medicine dealing with tumors or abnormal growths such as cancer.

Ophthalmologist — A medical doctor specializing in diseases of the eye.

Ophthalmoscope — An instrument for examining the eye.

Optometrist — A licensed, nonmedical practitioner who specializes in the diagnosis and treatment of vision defects.

Oral — Pertaining to the mouth.

Originator — The person who writes a check to issue payment.

Orthodontics — The branch of dentistry dealing with prevention and correction of irregularities of the alignment of the teeth.

Orthopedics — Branch of medicine or surgery dealing with the treatment of diseases and deformities of bones, muscles, and joints.

Osteoporosis — Condition in which bones become porous and brittle due to a lack of or loss of calcium, phosphorus, and other minerals.

Otoscope — An instrument for examining the ear.

Papanicolaou test — A PAP test; a test to classify abnormal cells in the vagina or cervix.

Parenteral — Other than by mouth; usually refers to the injection of substances into the veins and subcutaneous tissues.

Pathogen —Disease-producing organism; a germ.

Pathology — The study of the cause or nature of a disease.

Payee — A person receiving payment.

Pediatrics — The branch of medicine dealing with the care and treatment of diseases and disorders of children.

pH — A measurement scale to determine the degree of acidity or alkalinity of a substance.

Phalanges — Bones of the fingers and toes.

Pharmacology — The science that deals with the study of drugs.

Phlebotomist — An individual who collects blood and prepares it for tests.

Physical therapy — Treatment by physical means such as heat, cold, water, massage, or electricity.

Physician — A medical doctor.

Physician's Desk Reference (PDR) — A reference book that contains essential information on drugs and medications.

Physiology — The study of the processes or functions of living organisms.

Plasma — The liquid portion of blood.

Postoperative — Care given after surgery.

Postpartum — The period following delivery of a baby.

Prenatal — Before birth.

Preoperative — Care given before surgery.

Prophylactic — Preventative; an agent that prevents disease.

Protozoa — Microscopic one-celled animals often found in decayed materials and contaminated water.

Psychology — The study of mental processes and their effects on behavior.

Pulse — Pressure of the blood felt against the wall of an artery as the heart contracts or beats.

Pulse deficit — The difference between the rate of an apical pulse and the rate of a radial pulse.

Radiology — The branch of medicine dealing with X rays and radioactive substances.

Rate — The number per minute as used with pulse and respiration counts.

Reagent strip — Special test strips with chemical substances that react to the presence of other substances in urine or blood.

Receipt — A written record that money or goods has been received.

Rectum — Lower part of the large intestine that serves as a temporary storage area for indigestibles.

Refractometer — An instrument used to measure specific gravity of urine.

Respiration — Process of taking in oxygen (inspiration) and expelling carbon dioxide (expiration) by the lungs and air passages.

Restoration — The process of replacing a diseased portion of a tooth or a lost tooth by artificial means.

Rickettsiae — Parasitic microorganisms that live on another living organism.

Rubber base — Dental impression material that is elastic and rubbery in nature.

Smear — Material spread thinly on a slide for microscopic examination.

Specific gravity — The weight or mass of a substance compared with an equal amount of another substance used as a standard.

Sphygmomanometer — An instrument calibrated for measuring blood pressure in millimeters of mercury.

Sputum — Substance coughed up from the bronchi.

Sterile — Free of all organisms including spores and viruses.

Stethoscope — An instrument for listening to internal body sounds.

Stool — Material evacuated from the intestines; feces.

Subcutaneous — Injected or inserted beneath or under the skin.

Sublingual — Under the tongue.

Technician — An individual who meets a level of proficiency that usually requires a two-year associate degree or three to four years of on-the-job training.

Technologist — An individual who meets a level of proficiency that usually requires at least three to four years of college plus work experience.

Temperature — A measurement of the balance between heat lost and heat produced by the body.

Therapy — The remedial treatment of a disease or disorder.

Thermometer — An instrument used for measuring temperature.

Ultrasonic unit — A piece of equipment that cleans with high-frequency sound waves.

Urinary drainage unit — A special device consisting of tubing and a collection container that is connected to a urinary catheter to collect urine.

Urinary sediments — Solid materials suspended in urine.

Urine — Fluid excreted by the kidney.

Urinometer — A calibrated device used to measure specific gravity of urine.

Urology — The science dealing with urine and diseases of the urinary tract.

Vaccine — A substance given to an individual to produce immunity to a disease.

Venipuncture — Surgical puncture of a vein; inserting a needle into a vein.

Veterinary — Medical treatment of diseases or injuries to animals.

Virus — A large group of very small microorganisms, many of which cause disease.

Vital signs — Determinations that provide information about body conditions; includes temperature, pulse, respiration, and blood pressure measurements.

Vitamins — Organic substances necessary for body processes and life.

Void — To empty the urinary bladder or urinate.

Vomit — To expel material from the stomach and/or intestine through the mouth and/or nose.

ANSWERS TO ODD-NUMBERED PROBLEMS

SECTION 1   WHOLE NUMBERS

UNIT 1   ADDITION OF WHOLE NUMBERS

1. a. 419
   c. 14,068
   e. 7,422
3. 58
5. $131
7. 2,510 ml

9. 373 mg
11. 1,315 cc
13. 2,872 mg
15. a. $291,281
    c. $412,525

UNIT 2   SUBTRACTION OF WHOLE NUMBERS

1. a. 286
   c. 80,344
   e. 531,408
3. 8 cm
5. 34 hours
7. $2,138

9. $448
11. 65 degrees
13. a. 90 lb
    c. molars and incisors
15. a. $70,709

UNIT 3   MULTIPLICATION OF WHOLE NUMBERS

1. Multiplication Table

0	1	2	3	4	5	6	7	8	9
1	1	2	3	4	5	6	7	8	9
2	2	4	6	8	10	12	14	16	18
3	3	6	9	12	15	18	21	24	27
4	4	8	12	16	20	24	28	32	36
5	5	10	15	20	25	30	35	40	45
6	6	12	18	24	30	36	42	48	54
7	7	14	21	28	35	42	49	56	63
8	8	16	24	32	40	48	56	64	72
9	9	18	27	36	45	54	63	72	81

3. 720 cc
5. a. 750 ml
7. 56
9. 70
11. 390 oz

13. Beers 2,355 cal
    Smith 3,135 cal
    Webel 3,300 cal
15. $19,440
17. 227,395

UNIT 4   DIVISION OF WHOLE NUMBERS

1. a. 42
   c. 108
   e. 104 R 221
3. $37
5. $1,879

7. 45 pipettes
9. $2,157
11. 5 glasses
13. $19
15. 47 gm

UNIT 5   COMBINED OPERATIONS WITH WHOLE NUMBERS

1. a. 96
   b. 309
   e. 120
3. 1,980 cc
5. $16 hemostat
7. 26 oz
9. a. 8 breaths

11. 6,100
13. 9 cans
15. $17,480
17. $1,664
19. 25
21. a. 105,100
    c. 215,900

SECTION 2   COMMON FRACTIONS

UNIT 6   ADDITION OF COMMON FRACTIONS

1. a. $9/8$ or $1\frac{1}{8}$
   c. $4\frac{1}{2}$
   e. $67\frac{19}{40}$
3. $1\frac{3}{16}$ in
5. $4\frac{1}{4}$ miles

7. $11\frac{3}{4}$ lb
9. $26\frac{1}{4}$ minutes
11. a. no
13. $\frac{7}{24}$ gr
15. $2\frac{17}{24}$ oz

UNIT 7   SUBTRACTION OF COMMON FRACTIONS

1. a. $9/16$
   c. $4 9/16$
   e. $48 29/40$
3. $4 1/2$ gm
5. $241 3/4$ lb
7. 8 in

9. $1/15$ second
11. $2 9/16$ in
13. a. $11 3/4$ picocuries
15. a. Atlantic and Gulf Coastal Plain
    c. $1 7/20$ mSv

UNIT 8   MULTIPLICATION OF COMMON FRACTIONS

1. a. $9/32$
   c. $48 1/3$
   e. $1,450 2/9$
3. 38
5. $1/8$ gr
7. 10 mAs

9. 750 mg
11. 22,293
13. a. $3 3/4$ hours
    c. $1 7/8$ hours
15. 10 mAs
17. $467,698

UNIT 9   DIVISION OF COMMON FRACTIONS

1. a. $1 1/20$
   c. $10 1/2$
   e. $1/80$
3. $13 1/2$ doses
5. 137 semester hours

7. 250,000
9. 1,500 ml
11. 20,648
13. a. $450
15. 1,500 cc

UNIT 10   COMBINED OPERATIONS WITH COMMON FRACTIONS

1. a. $5/8$
   c. $23/46$
3. a. $18 3/4$ oz
5. 895 cc
7. a. no
9. a. $1/2$ lb
   c. $3/4$ lb

11. $5 1/3$ days
13. a. $11/32$
    c. 7,515
15. a. 63,205,000
    c. 28,442,250
17. 213,560,000
19. a. $4/9$

SECTION 3   DECIMAL FRACTIONS

UNIT 11   ADDITION OF DECIMAL FRACTIONS

1. a. 93.713
   c. 511.282
   e. 5509.559
3. 7.75 hours
5. $2,708.49
7. 48.5 mAs

9. $322.54
11. 0.736 gm
13. a. 10.8 gm
    c. 42.3 gm
15. 8.43472 l
17. 0.075 mg

UNIT 12   SUBTRACTION OF DECIMAL FRACTIONS

1. a. 28.76
   c. 91.71
   e. 89.78
3. $2,514.78
5. 0.015
7. 3.8°F

9. 4.5 gm
11. a. less, 0.0001
13. 1.6
15. $69,855.84
17. 17.07 million

UNIT 13   MULTIPLICATION OF DECIMAL FRACTIONS

1. a. 229.732
   c. 0.097
   e. 0.003
3. 10.8 gm
5. 3 sec
7. 18.502 lb

9. 390.5 cal
11. 30 mAs
13. $111.36
15. 43,908,520 to 46,251,620
17. 236,600 to 405,600

UNIT 14   DIVISION OF DECIMAL FRACTIONS

1. a. 53.4
   c. 11,142.85714 or 11,142.86
   e. 144.3410093 or 144.34
3. $14.33
5. 0.679 lb
7. $11.53

9. 140
11. a. 107
13. $108.90 for 36 exposures
15. 1.25 gr
17. 2 ml

UNIT 15 DECIMAL AND COMMON FRACTION EQUIVALENTS

1. a. 0.313
   c. 43.6
3. $98\frac{3}{5}$
5. °F = $\frac{9}{5}$ °C + 32
7. a. $\frac{1}{10}$
9. a. $\frac{3}{25}$
   c. $\frac{1}{20}$
   e. $\frac{2}{25}$
   g. $\frac{1}{10}$

11. 146 doses
13. 3.977 kg
15. $1\frac{1}{2}$ tablets
17. a. bacterium

UNIT 16 COMBINED OPERATIONS WITH DECIMAL FRACTIONS

1. a. 2.164
   c. 8.091
3. $3,554.03
5. $219.70
7. $621.60
9. $149.66

11. $153.37
13. a. 468 cal
15. 14 students at $0.41/student
17. a. 0.09 gm
    c. 0.16125 gm
19. $2,580.27 or $2,580.28

SECTION 4 PERCENT, INTEREST, AND AVERAGES

UNIT 17 PERCENT AND PERCENTAGE

1. a. 0.39
   c. $\frac{13}{20}$
   e. 0.004
3. 3,147.12
5. 10.4 oz
7. a. 587.88
   c. 75.02
9. a. $45,716.58
11. a. 28.4%
    c. 242.95

13. 4,410.69
15. a. 85%
    c. 241,834.12
17. $535.44
19. 82,020,327.84
21. 3
23. 75%

UNIT 18 INTEREST AND DISCOUNTS

1. a. $756.00
3. a. $44.10
5. $3,926.56
7. a. Super Price
9. a. $84,233.19
   c. $4,185.21

11. $5,842.95
13. 46.24%
15. $4,069.81
17. $389.20
19. $241.49

UNIT 19 AVERAGES AND ESTIMATES

1. a. 47.8
   c. 83.2%
   e. 31³⁄₁₀ in or 31.3 in
3. a. 30%
5. a. 2,335.57 mg
7. a. 119.5 mg
9. 101

11. 83°F
13. 720 or 735
15. 96.5%
17. $65,575.86
19. a. 5,760
    c. 336.96 or 337
21. $463.55

SECTION 5 RATIO AND PROPORTION

UNIT 20 RATIO

1. a. 1 to 3, 1:3, or ⅓
   c. 2 to 1, 2:1, or ²⁄₁
3. 1 to 20 or 1:20
5. 12 to 43 or 12:43
7. a. 2 to 7 or 2:7
   c. 1 to 2.5 or 1:2.5

9. 44 to 297 or 1 to 6.75
11. 1 to 10 rem
13. $4,620,000
15. 1 to 51.43 or 1:51.43
17. 50 ml

UNIT 21 PROPORTION

1. a. 900 mg
   c. 60 ml
3. 45 ml
5. 35 mm
7. 10 gm

9. 5 ml
11. a. $235.65
13. 0.14 to 0.24 parts
15. ½ ml or 0.5 ml
17. a. 41 hours

SECTION 6   METRIC AND OTHER MEASUREMENTS

UNIT 22   LINEAR MEASUREMENT

1. a. 8,450.0 m
   c. 34,320.0 m
   e. 54.68 m
3. 0.9712 mm
5. a. bacterium

7. 1,800 mm
9. $0.61
11. a. 0.4953 m
13. 12-cm pipette
15. 176.10 cm

UNIT 23   MASS OR WEIGHT MEASUREMENT

1. a. 7,563.0 gm
   c. 560 gm
   e. 0.00921 gm
3. 3.178 kg
5. 4.6875 or 4 crackers
7. a. 612.204 gm
   c. 123,240.8 mg

9. 82.628 kg
11. a. 375 mg
13. 25%
15. a. 25.310 or 25.341 kg
    c. 3 ml

UNIT 24   VOLUME OR LIQUID MEASUREMENT

1. a. 5.6923 l
   c. 8.82 l
   e. 5.185 l
3. 6.7
5. 50
7. 1 ml or 0.1 cl

9. a. 50 mg
11. 5 to 6 qt
13. a. 36 ml
15. a. 15 ml
    c. 5 ml

UNIT 25   CELSIUS AND FAHRENHEIT

1. 15°C
3. 4.4°C or 4.5°C
5. 28°C
7. 50°F
9. 119.66°F or 119.7°F

11. 98.6°F
13. 114.98°F or 115°F
15. 95°F
17. 2.5°C

UNIT 26 ROMAN NUMERALS

1. XXVII
3. XCIV
5. MMDCXLVIII
7. 86

9. 1,994
11. 2 tablets
13. 1947
15. a. MMMXXVIII

UNIT 27 APOTHECARIES' SYSTEM

1. a. 1.4 gm
  c. 8 tbsp
  e. 45 gtt
  g. 0.0075 gm
3. 1 dram
5. ¼ oz

7. a. 150 ml
9. 90 mg
11. 2 tablets
13. 2 ml
15. 4 tablets
17. a. ½ ml

SECTION 7 MEASUREMENT INSTRUMENTS

UNIT 28 RULERS OR TAPE MEASURES

1. 3⅛ in
3. 5⅝ in
5. 9¼ in
7. 41 in
9. 45¾ in

11. 58½ in
13. 69¾ in
15. 3 ft 2 in
17. 4 ft 5½ in
19. 5 ft 7¾ in

UNIT 29 SCALES

1. 103 lb
3. 109¼ lb
5. 124½ lb
7. 256¾ lb
9. 269½ lb

11. 1 lb 6 oz
13. 3 lb 10 oz
15. 5 lb 7 oz
17. 4 lb 4½ oz
19. 9 lb 10¼ oz

UNIT 30 THERMOMETERS

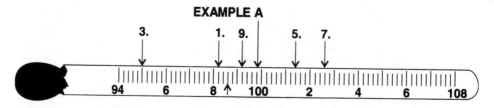

EXAMPLE A

11. 95.6°

13. 98.2°

15. 100.4°

17. 103°

19. 105.8°

UNIT 31   SPHYGMOMANOMETER GAUGES

1. 276

3. 218

5. 164

7. 94

9. 64

11. 250

13. 214

15. 154

17. 116

19. 74

UNIT 32   SYRINGES

1. 0.4 or ⅖ ml

3. 2 ml

5. 5 m

7. 24 m

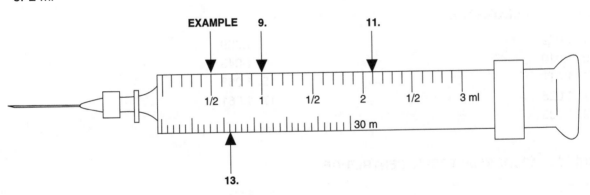

15. 0.1 or ¹⁄₁₀ ml

17. 0.53 or ⁵³⁄₁₀₀ ml

19. 0.86 or ²¹⁄₂₅ ml

21. 7 m

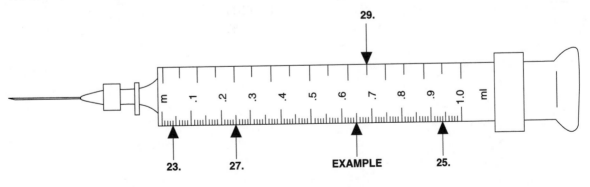

31. 7 U

33. 34 U

35. 16 U

37. 68 U

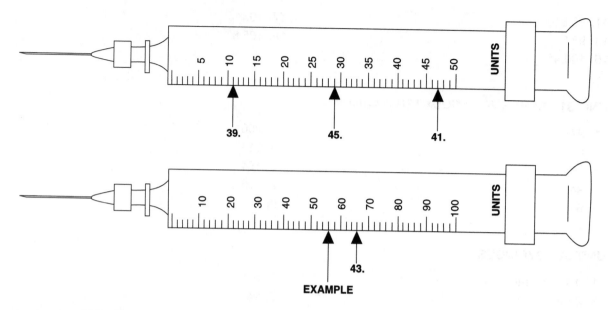

UNIT 33   URINOMETER

1. 1.002
3. 1.010
5. 1.017
7. 1.025
9. 1.033

11. 1.039
13. 1.045
15. 1.053
17. 1.061

UNIT 34   MICROHEMATOCRIT CENTRIFUGE

1. 5%
3. 13%
5. 22%
7. 28%
9. 34%

11. 43%
13. 49%
15. 58%
17. 65%
19. 77%

SECTION 8 GRAPHS AND CHARTS

UNIT 35 TEMPERATURE, PULSE, AND RESPIRATION (TPR) GRAPHICS

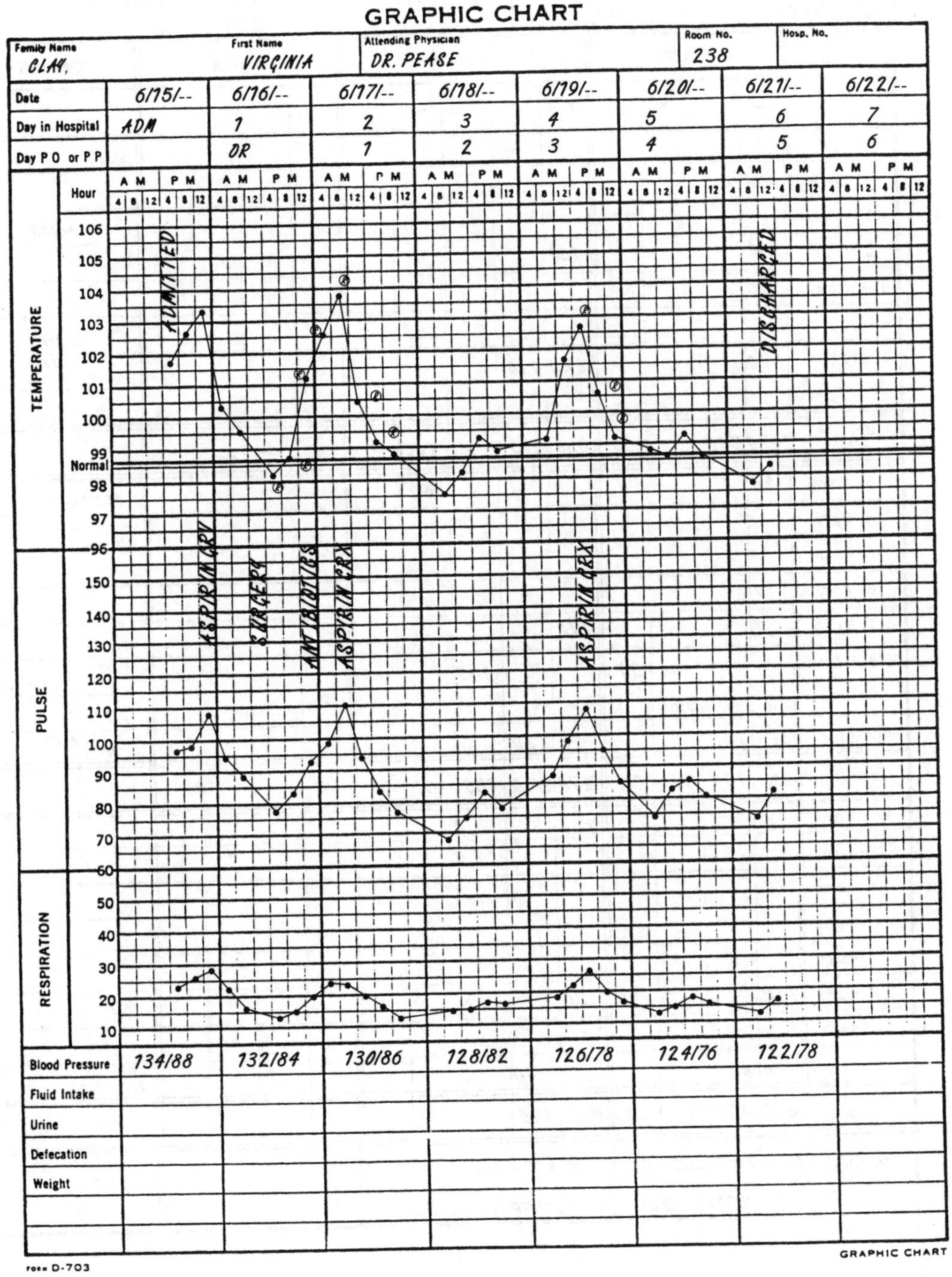

GRAPHIC CHART

GRAPHIC CHART

ross D-703

UNIT 36   INTAKE AND OUTPUT CHARTS

<table>
<tr><td colspan="16" align="center">INTAKE AND OUTPUT RECORD</td></tr>
<tr>
<td colspan="5">Family Name
BARTLETT</td>
<td colspan="4">First Name
DENNIS</td>
<td colspan="2">Attending Physician</td>
<td colspan="2">Room No.
238</td>
<td colspan="3">Hosp. No.</td>
</tr>
<tr>
<td>Date
9/30</td>
<td colspan="4" align="center">INTAKE</td>
<td colspan="4" align="center">OUTPUT</td>
<td colspan="4" align="center">OTHER</td>
<td colspan="2" align="center">REMARKS</td>
</tr>
<tr>
<td>TIME</td>
<td>Oral</td><td>I.V.</td><td>Blood</td><td>N/G</td>
<td>Urine</td><td>Tube</td><td>Emesis</td><td>Feces</td>
<td></td><td></td><td></td><td></td>
<td colspan="2"></td>
</tr>
<tr><td>7 - 8 a.m.</td><td>240</td><td></td><td></td><td></td><td>230</td><td></td><td></td><td></td><td></td><td></td><td></td><td></td><td colspan="2"></td></tr>
<tr><td>8 - 9 a.m.</td><td>560</td><td></td><td></td><td></td><td></td><td></td><td></td><td></td><td></td><td></td><td></td><td></td><td colspan="2"></td></tr>
<tr><td>9 - 10 a.m.</td><td></td><td></td><td></td><td>10</td><td></td><td></td><td></td><td></td><td></td><td></td><td></td><td></td><td colspan="2" rowspan="3" align="center">NG/NS</td></tr>
<tr><td>10 - 11 a.m.</td><td>240</td><td></td><td></td><td></td><td>180</td><td></td><td></td><td></td><td></td><td></td><td></td><td></td></tr>
<tr><td>11 - 12 noon</td><td>580</td><td></td><td></td><td></td><td></td><td></td><td></td><td></td><td></td><td></td><td></td><td></td></tr>
<tr><td>12 - 1 p.m.</td><td></td><td></td><td></td><td></td><td></td><td></td><td>260</td><td></td><td></td><td></td><td></td><td></td><td colspan="2">EMESIS-
LT. BROWN</td></tr>
<tr><td>1 - 2 p.m.</td><td>540</td><td></td><td></td><td></td><td>220</td><td>770</td><td></td><td></td><td></td><td></td><td></td><td></td><td colspan="2">NG/CLEAR
NG/LT. YELLOW</td></tr>
<tr><td>2 - 3 p.m.</td><td></td><td></td><td></td><td></td><td></td><td></td><td></td><td></td><td></td><td></td><td></td><td></td><td colspan="2"></td></tr>
<tr><td>8 HOUR
TOTAL</td><td>1620</td><td>540</td><td></td><td>10</td><td>630</td><td>770</td><td></td><td>260</td><td></td><td></td><td></td><td></td><td colspan="2"></td></tr>
<tr><td>3 - 4 p.m.</td><td>120</td><td></td><td></td><td></td><td></td><td></td><td>160</td><td></td><td></td><td></td><td></td><td></td><td colspan="2">FECES-LT. BROWN</td></tr>
<tr><td>4 - 5 p.m.</td><td></td><td></td><td></td><td></td><td></td><td></td><td></td><td></td><td></td><td></td><td></td><td></td><td colspan="2"></td></tr>
<tr><td>5 - 6 p.m.</td><td></td><td></td><td></td><td></td><td></td><td></td><td></td><td></td><td></td><td></td><td></td><td></td><td colspan="2"></td></tr>
<tr><td>6 - 7 p.m.</td><td>510</td><td></td><td></td><td></td><td></td><td></td><td></td><td></td><td></td><td></td><td></td><td></td><td colspan="2"></td></tr>
<tr><td>7 - 8 p.m.</td><td></td><td></td><td></td><td></td><td>270</td><td></td><td></td><td></td><td></td><td></td><td></td><td></td><td colspan="2"></td></tr>
<tr><td>8 - 9 p.m.</td><td></td><td></td><td></td><td>30</td><td></td><td>180</td><td></td><td></td><td></td><td></td><td></td><td></td><td colspan="2">EMESIS-
LT. YELLOW</td></tr>
<tr><td>9 - 10 p.m.</td><td>45</td><td></td><td>500</td><td></td><td></td><td></td><td></td><td></td><td></td><td></td><td></td><td></td><td colspan="2">IV-BLOOD</td></tr>
<tr><td>10 - 11 p.m.</td><td>30</td><td>150</td><td></td><td></td><td></td><td>220</td><td></td><td></td><td></td><td></td><td></td><td></td><td colspan="2">NG/LT.-GOLD/BROWN
IV-NS</td></tr>
<tr><td>8 HOUR
TOTAL</td><td>705</td><td>150</td><td>500</td><td>30</td><td>270</td><td>220</td><td>180</td><td>160</td><td></td><td></td><td></td><td></td><td colspan="2"></td></tr>
<tr><td>11 - 12 p.m.</td><td>60</td><td></td><td></td><td></td><td>280</td><td></td><td></td><td></td><td></td><td></td><td></td><td></td><td colspan="2"></td></tr>
<tr><td>12 - 1 a.m.</td><td></td><td></td><td></td><td></td><td></td><td></td><td></td><td></td><td></td><td></td><td></td><td></td><td colspan="2"></td></tr>
<tr><td>1 - 2 a.m.</td><td>120</td><td></td><td></td><td></td><td></td><td></td><td></td><td></td><td></td><td></td><td></td><td></td><td colspan="2"></td></tr>
<tr><td>2 - 3 a.m.</td><td></td><td></td><td></td><td></td><td></td><td></td><td></td><td></td><td></td><td></td><td></td><td></td><td colspan="2"></td></tr>
<tr><td>3 - 4 a.m.</td><td></td><td></td><td></td><td></td><td></td><td></td><td></td><td></td><td></td><td></td><td></td><td></td><td colspan="2"></td></tr>
<tr><td>4 - 5 a.m.</td><td>240</td><td></td><td></td><td>20</td><td>180</td><td></td><td></td><td></td><td></td><td></td><td></td><td></td><td colspan="2" rowspan="2" align="center">NG/NS</td></tr>
<tr><td>5 - 6 a.m.</td><td></td><td></td><td></td><td></td><td></td><td></td><td></td><td></td><td></td><td></td><td></td><td></td></tr>
<tr><td>6 - 7 a.m.</td><td>180</td><td>450</td><td></td><td></td><td></td><td>140</td><td></td><td></td><td></td><td></td><td></td><td></td><td colspan="2">IV/NS
NG/LT. YELLOW</td></tr>
<tr><td>8 HOUR
TOTAL</td><td>600</td><td>450</td><td></td><td>20</td><td>460</td><td>140</td><td></td><td></td><td></td><td></td><td></td><td></td><td colspan="2"></td></tr>
<tr><td>24 HOUR
TOTAL</td><td>2925</td><td>1140</td><td>500</td><td>60</td><td>1360</td><td>470</td><td>440</td><td>160</td><td></td><td></td><td></td><td></td><td colspan="2"></td></tr>
<tr><td></td><td colspan="4">TOTAL INTAKE 4625</td><td colspan="4">TOTAL OUTPUT   2430</td><td></td><td></td><td></td><td></td><td colspan="2"></td></tr>
</table>

UNIT 37 HEIGHT/WEIGHT MEASUREMENT GRAPHS

Birth to 36 months: Girls
Length-for-age and Weight-for-age percentiles

NAME _____ Nartker, Kaleigh _____

RECORD # _____ 161142 _____

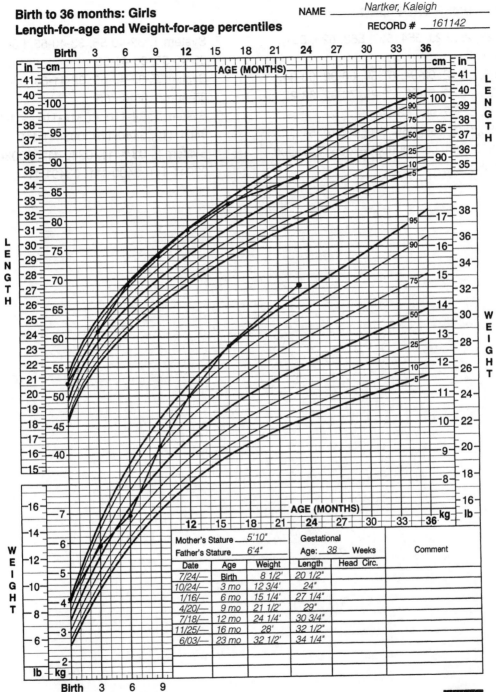

	Mother's Stature	5'10"		Gestational		
	Father's Stature	6'4"		Age: 38 Weeks		Comment
Date	Age	Weight	Length	Head Circ.		
7/24/—	Birth	8 1/2'	20 1/2"			
10/24/—	3 mo	12 3/4'	24"			
1/16/—	6 mo	15 1/4'	27 1/4"			
4/20/—	9 mo	21 1/2'	29"			
7/18/—	12 mo	24 1/4'	30 3/4"			
11/25/—	16 mo	28'	32 1/2"			
6/03/—	23 mo	32 1/2'	34 1/4"			

Published May 30, 2000 (modified 4/20/01).
SOURCE: Developed by the National Center for Health Statistics in collaboration with
the National Center for Chronic Disease Prevention and Health Promotion (2000).
http://www.cdc.gov/growthcharts

SAFER • HEALTHIER • PEOPLE™

SECTION 9   ACCOUNTING AND BUSINESS

UNIT 38 NUMERICAL FILING

1. 22, 23, 25, 523, 554, 567, 568, 829, 831, and 904

3. 00-56, 02-92, 02-94, 07-56, 08-92, 08-94, 71-25, 71-52, 71-92, 78-25, 78-92, 88-25, 88-92, 88-93, and 88-94

5. 05, 50, 051, 055, 056, 500, 00510, 511, 0543, 00553, 555, 0000556, 00571, 05000, and 05011

7. System 1: 32-40-55, 33-40-55, 56-41-55, 65-40-55, 65-41-55
   System 2: 32-40-65, 32-41-65, 64-41-65, 65-40-65, 65-65-65

9. System 1: 34-110, 00314-110, 341-110, 3401-110, 3440-110, 003441-110
   System 2: 034-111, 0340-111, 000341-111, 03041-111, 3400-111, 03401-111

UNIT 39   APPOINTMENT SCHEDULES

APPOINTMENT SCHEDULE

DATE: Monday, 00/00/00		DATE: Tuesday, 00/00/00	
8:30	Martin, Carol	8:30	Dental Board
8:45	Prophy and Fl	8:45	Meeting
9:00		9:00	
9:15	Beal, Jerry	9:15	
9:30	Extraction	9:30	
9:45	Feltner, Joyce	9:45	
10:00	Composite	10:00	Sheely Children–Mark & Mike
10:15	Wolf, Tom	10:15	Exam and Fl
10:30	Prophy and Exam	10:30	Purvis, Kelly
10:45		10:45	Composite
11:00	Barr, Shelly	11:00	Darbey, Nancy X-rays
11:15	Endodontic	11:15	Grandy, Tom
11:30		11:30	Prophy and Exam
11:45		11:45	
12:00		12:00	
12:15	Lunch	12:15	Lunch
12:30		12:30	
12:45		12:45	
1:00	Carey, Karen Crown	1:00	Holmes, Ed
1:15	Knowlton, Linda	1:15	Amalgam
1:30	Composite	1:30	Tenney, Tom
1:45		1:45	Endodontics
2:00	Frank, Jackie	2:00	
2:15	Crown	2:15	
2:30		2:30	
2:45	Bush, Phil	2:45	
3:00	Amalgam	3:00	Berry, Dave
3:15	Schultheis, Kathy	3:15	Amalgam
3:30	Extraction	3:30	Mock Children: Tom, Trevor, Tim
3:45		3:45	Prophy and Fl
4:00		4:00	
4:15		4:15	
4:30	Cooper, Randal Crown	4:30	

UNIT 40   CALCULATING CASH TRANSACTIONS

1.

	Say $32.00
Give $1.00	Say $33.00
Give $1.00	Say $34.00
Give $1.00	Say $35.00
Give $5.00	Say $40.00
Give $10.00	Say $50.00

3.

	Say $12.65
Give $0.10	Say $12.75
Give $0.25	Say $13.00
Give $1.00	Say $14.00
Give $1.00	Say $15.00

5.

	Say $65.85
Give $0.05	Say $65.90
Give $0.10	Say $66.00
Give $1.00	Say $67.00
Give $1.00	Say $68.00
Give $1.00	Say $69.00
Give $1.00	Say $70.00
Give $10.00	Say $80.00
Give $20.00	Say $100.00

7.

	Say $43.58
Give $0.01	Say $43.59
Give $0.01	Say $43.60
Give $0.05	Say $43.65
Give $0.10	Say $43.75
Give $0.25	Say $44.00
Give $1.00	Say $45.00
Give $5.00	Say $50.00
Give $10.00	Say $60.00

9.

	Say $105.55
Give $0.10	Say $105.65
Give $0.10	Say $105.75
Give $0.25	Say $106.00
Give $1.00	Say $107.00
Give $1.00	Say $108.00
Give $1.00	Say $109.00
Give $1.00	Say $110.00

11. **Date:** ___10/11/-- ___

NUMBER	DENOMINATION		AMOUNT
45	Pennies	(× .01)	.45
132	Nickles	(× .05)	6.60
92	Dimes	(× .10)	9.20
136	Quarters	(× .25)	34.00
7	Half-Dollars	(× .50)	3.50
61	$1 Bills	(× 1.00)	61.00
22	$5 Bills	(× 5.00)	110.00
18	$10 Bills	(× 10.00)	180.00
12	$20 Bills	(× 20.00)	240.00
3	$50 Bills	(× 50.00)	150.00
2	$100 Bills	(× 100.00)	200.00
	TOTAL AMOUNT		994.75

Beginning Cash Balance	50.00
+ Total of Cash Payments	944.75
TOTAL	994.75
- Payments Made From Cash Drawer	—
FINAL CASH AMOUNT	994.75

a. $994.75   b. yes

UNIT 41   MAINTAINING ACCOUNTS

1. $24.00   7. a. $1,298.96
3. $202.11   9. $221.71
5. $161.60   11. $147.09

13.

DATE	PATIENT NAME	TREATMENT	CHARGE		PAYMENT		CURRENT BALANCE	
3/25/--	Steidl, Sue	OV	68	50	25	00	43	50
4/14/--	Steidl, Sue	OV, Bl Tests	125	90	35	50	133	90
5/28/--	Steidl, Sue	OV, ECG	171	25	48	50	256	65
6/2/--	Steidl, Sue	OV, Meds	135	68	—	—	392	33
6/9/--	Steidl, Sue	ROA-Insurance	—	—	356	37	35	96

15.

DATE	PATIENT NAME	TREATMENT	CHARGE		PAYMENT		CURRENT BALANCE	
		Previous Balance					586	33
10/11/--	Lichtner, Pat	Sp XR-4, SpMan-1/2	203	25	25	50	764	08
10/19/--	Lichtner, Pat	SpMan-3/4	48	38	25	50	786	96
11/02/--	Lichtner, Pat	Acup-1/2, Sp XR-2	127	80	34	75	880	01
11/08/--	Lichtner, Pat	HCPk, SpMan-1/4	57	83	—	—	937	84
11/10/--	Lichtner, Pat	ROA-Insurance	—	—	428	64	509	20
11/16/--	Lichtner, Pat	SpMan-3/4, Acup-1/3	76	58	48	75	537	03

UNIT 42   CHECKS, DEPOSIT SLIPS, AND RECEIPTS

1.

No. _1_ $ _232 68/100_	Happy Doctor, MD	No. ___1___	
Date _7/12_ 20__	1 Healthy Lane		
To _ILLUMINATING_	Fitness, OH 11133	_JULY 1_ 20__	
For _____			

Pay to the Order of: __ILLUMINATING COMPANY__ $232 68/100

TWO HUNDRED THIRTY-TWO AND 68/100 ———— Dollars

Balance	1014	34
Am't Dep.	—	—
Total	1014	34
Am't Ck.	232	68
Balance	781	66

First Money Bank
1 Rich Lane
Wealthy, OH 11133
00098-5567   By _____
Memo _ELECTRIC_

3.

Happy Doctor, M.D.
1 Healthy Lane
Fitness, OH 11133

Date _____ _JULY 1_ _____ 20 —

Signature _____
                (If cash received)

First Money Bank
1 Rich Lane
Wealthy, OH 11133
0098-5567

Currency	648	00
Coin	52	73
Checks	76	42
	321	68
	159	20
TOTAL	1258	03
Less Cash	—	—
TOTAL DEPOSIT	1258	03

5.

No. _____1_____	No. ___1___	JULY 1 20 ___
Date ___7/1/--___	Received From _____JAMES JOHNSON_____	
To __J. JOHNSON__	ONE HUNDRED FIFTY-SIX AND $^{90}\!/_{100}$ ————— Dollars	
For _____POA_____	For _POA-PHYSICAL EXAM_	
Amount _$156 $^{90}\!/_{100}$_	$ 156 $^{90}\!/_{100}$ *Louise Simmers*	

7. Answers not included since this is a sequence of events. Use the samples shown in the text to complete the assignment. The final current balance in the account should be $454.04.

UNIT 43   PAYCHECK CALCULATION

1. $305.28
3. $959.40
5. a. $41.04
  c. $54.76
7. $302.45

9. $229.63
11. $288.75
13. $266.69
15. $437.18

17.

TIME AND SALARY COMPUTATION RECORD

Name _____   SS _____   Date _____

Marital Status *M*   Dependents *2*   Pay Rate *$9.13*

DATES	ON	OFF	HOURS	PAY CALCULATION	AMOUNTS	
12/08/–	*6 AM*	*3 PM*	*9*	Regular Pay: *40 x 9.13*	*365*	*20*
12/09/–	*6 AM*	*3 PM*	*9*	Overtime Pay: *9 x 1.5 x 9.13*	*123*	*26*
12/10/–	*8 AM*	*6 PM*	*10*	**TOTAL GROSS WAGES**	*488*	*46*
12/11/–				Deductions:		
12/12/–	*7 AM*	*3 PM*	*8*	Federal Withholding Tax	*40*	*14*
12/13/–	*6 AM*	*3 PM*	*9*	State Tax: 3%	*14*	*65*
12/14/–	*7 AM*	*11 AM*	*4*	City Tax: 2.5%	*12*	*21*
				FICA: 7.65%	*37*	*37*
				Other:		
				TOTAL DEDUCTIONS	*104*	*37*
TOTALS	**BASE:** *40*	**OT:** *9*		**AMOUNT OF CHECK**	*384*	*09*

SECTION 10   MATH FOR MEDICATIONS

UNIT 44 CALCULATING ORAL DOSAGE

1. 2 tablets
3. ½ tablet
5. 3 tablets
7. 1 ml
9. 2 tablets

11. 2½ ml
13. ½ tablet
15. 9 tsp
17. ½ tablet
19. gr ⅓

UNIT 45 CALCULATING PARENTERAL DOSAGE

1. 1½ ml or 1.5 ml
3. ½ ml or 0.5 ml
5. 10 ml
7. 1¼ or 1.25 ml
9. 1.5 or 1½ ml

11. 1.5 ml or 1½ ml
13. a. 10 ml
15. a. ¾ or 0.75 gm
17. 20 mg
19. 2 ml

UNIT 46   CALCULATING DOSAGE BY WEIGHT

1. a. 240 mg
3. a. 600 mg
5. a. 5,640 mg
7. a. 150 mg
9. a. 500 mg

11. a. 250 mg
13. a. 920 to 2,760 mg
15. a. 55.9 or 56 mg
17. a. no
19. 1.2 to 1.3 ml

UNIT 47   CALCULATING PEDIATRIC DOSAGE

1. a. yes
3. a. 118 to 177 mg
5. a. 19.1 to 38.25 mg
   c. 36 mg
7. a. 618 to 1236 mg
   c. 8 ml

9. a. 158,824 U with 0.45 m^2 BSA
11. a. 144 mg with 0.98 m^2 BSA
13. a. 0.147 gm with 0.5 m^2 BSA
15. a. 112.94 mg with 0.16 m^2 BSA
17. a. 14–28 units
19. a. 780 mg

UNIT 48   CALCULATING INTRAVENOUS FLOW RATES

1. 16.66 or 17 gtt/min
3. 50 gtt/min
5. 13.88 or 14 gtt/min
7. 31.25 or 31 gtt/min
9. 80 gtt/min
11. 50 hours

13. 0.56 hours or 33.3 minutes
15. a. 62.5 or 63 gtt/min
17. 360 ml
19. 558 ml
21. 14.6 or 15 gtt/min

UNIT 49   PREPARING AND DILUTING SOLUTIONS

1. 10 ml
3. 50 gm
5. 0.7875 gm
7. 24 ml
9. 7.5 ml
11. a. 9.75 gm

13. 116.67 or 117 ml
15. 145.83 or 146 ml
17. 28.72 or 29 ml
19. a. 0.6%
    c. 0.02%
21. 20 ml